T0352627

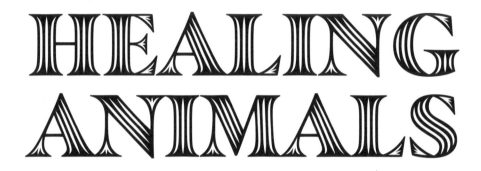

HEALING ANIMALS

Wolves, Foxes, Owls, and Other Wild Archetypal Animals
that Inhabit Our Psyche

Publisher
Balthazar Pagani

Graphic design and layout
Due mani non bastano

Vivida

Vivida® trademark is the property of White Star s.r.l.
www.vividabooks.com

© 2023 White Star s.r.l.
Piazzale Luigi Cadorna, 6
20123 Milano, Italia
www.whitestar.it

Translation: Contextus s.r.l., Italy (Flavia Frauzel)
Editing: Phillip Gaskill

ISBN 978-88-544-2038-0
1 2 3 4 5 6   27 26 25 24 23

Printed in China

Federica Zizzari Kikosmica

HEALING ANIMALS

Wolves, Foxes, Owls, and Other Wild Archetypal Animals
that Inhabit Our Psyche

Illustrations by Giada Ungredda

Vivida

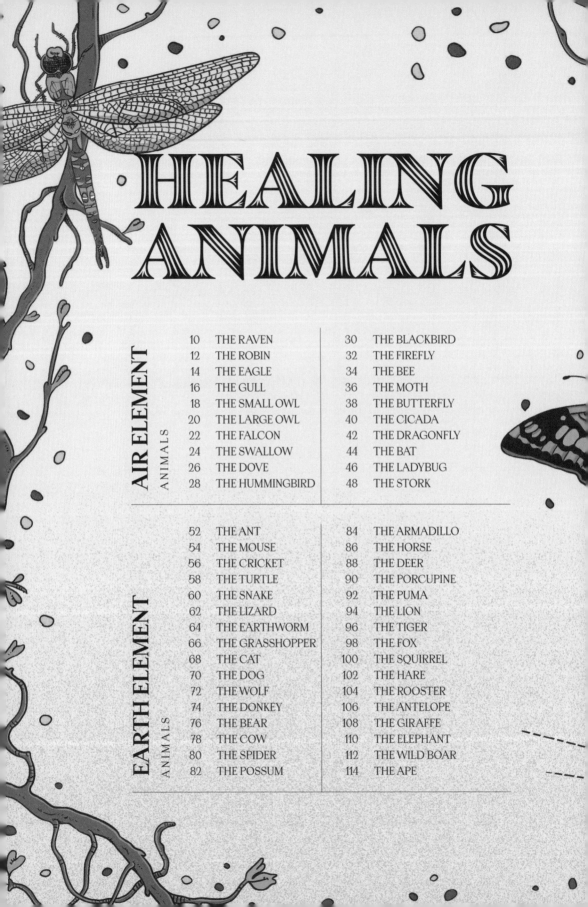

HEALING ANIMALS

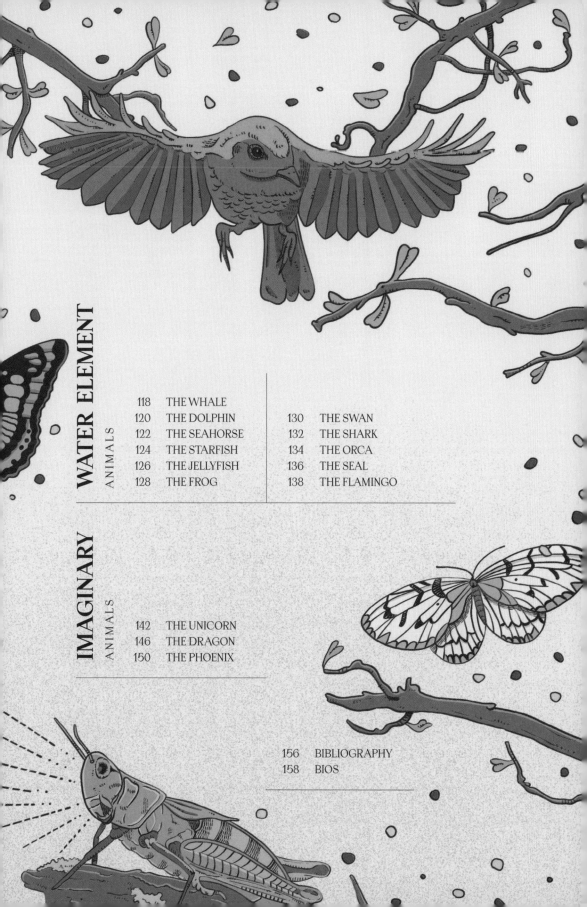

WATER ELEMENT
ANIMALS

IMAGINARY
ANIMALS

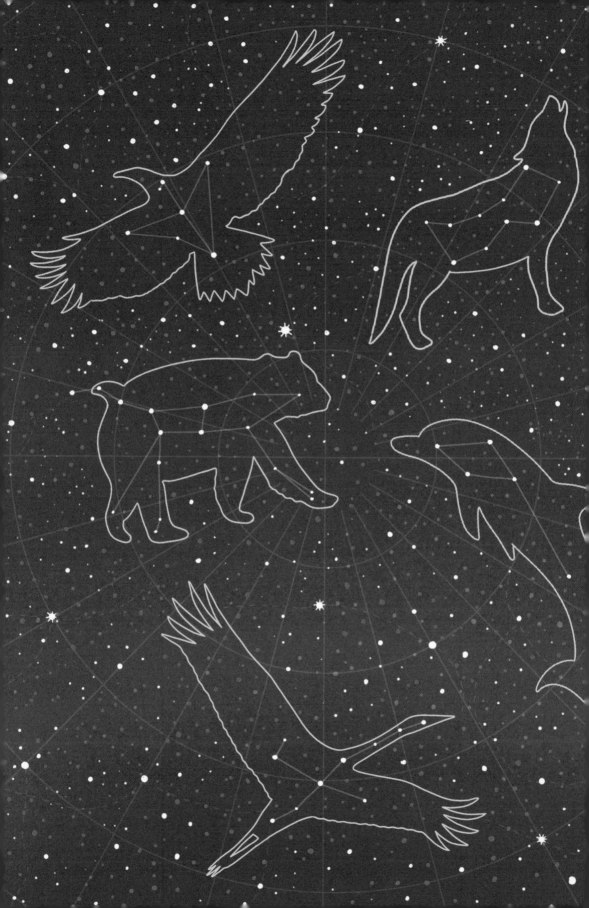

As human beings, we are children of the Earth, we have an animal nature that expresses itself through our body and a divine soul nature that is one with it. The animals we are going to discover and meet in this book represent—with their intrinsic attributes, which I like to call medicine—the inner resources we can access. Each power-enhancing animal embodies a unique and special medicine, a gift offered to the world from which we can draw energy, retrieving those gifts within us, so that they become useful tools for dealing with daily challenges. Precious mirrors in which we can recognize ourselves, discovering various parts of our being which we can add to, welcome, and love. If we understand their medicinal power, we will then know at which times we can harness it, to move together relying on the strength of an ally that will support and guide us through the process we are going through. Each of us has at least one power-bringing animal that accompanies us on our earthly journey, a precious guide that walks by our side, sometimes called an animal spirit, sometimes a totem animal. Certain of these accompany us throughout Life, others only for short periods. They are magical animals that make their energy force available so we can draw on it, enabling us to recognize our own energy force. These animal spirits have populated fables, fairy tales, myths, and legends from time immemorial, revealing their aspects of light and darkness; they have always moved us, at times frightened us, and, on other occasions, they have opened our Heart. They live in our daily life as well as in our psyche; and during the journey you are about to embark on you will learn to love them, marveling at how each of them will reveal a part of your being.

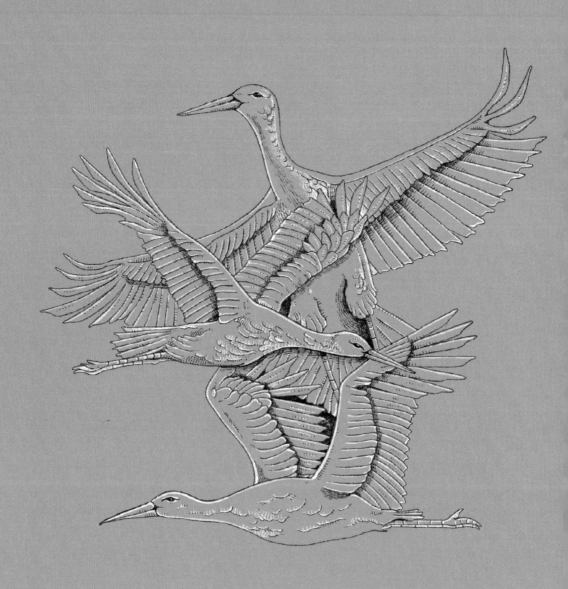

AIR ELEMENT ANIMALS

Air Element Animals shepherd us with their agility, creating space within us and conveying new perspectives. They open us to the possibility of flying, of seeing everything from above, of having high, wide, and open perspectives. They bring us closer to the reality of our Soul, placing the accent on the intangible aspect of flight. They are essential for reminding us that we can be something else, that our existence is not contained in the possibilities that our body offers us. They remind us of our Spirit's potential.

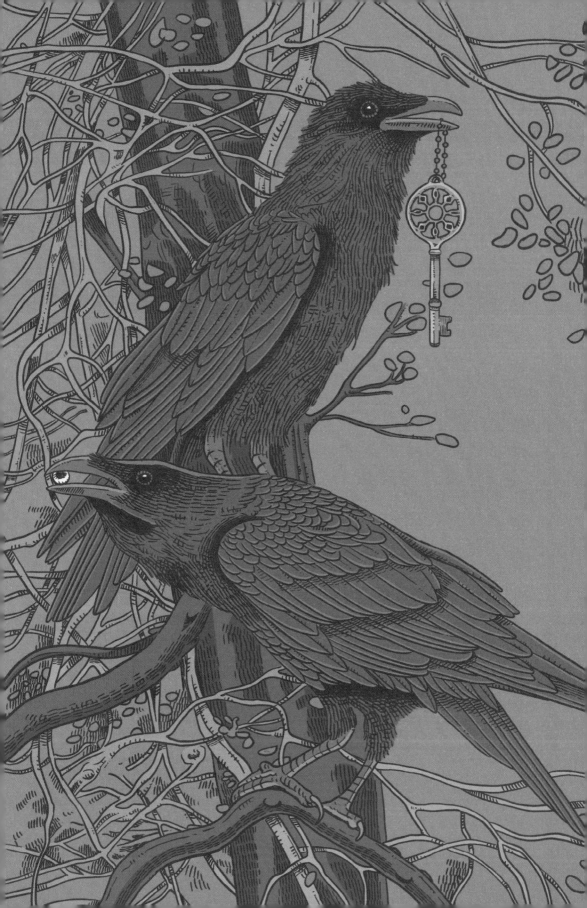

THE RAVEN
The Custodian of Magic

Black as midnight, the Raven is a farsighted, prophetic, and visionary animal. It is the messenger of emptiness, the primordial womb from which we all come, and in whose surrender we experience healing. Always associated with death, for its propensity for feeding on lifeless bodies, it is a fearsome initiatory bird, which soars over change, squawking at the transit between a cycle of death and one of rebirth. This coal-colored feathered friend brings us a powerful medicine as a gift. Not surprisingly, it is sacred to many deities, such as the two Ravens belonging to Odin, Muninn, "memory," and Huginn, "thought," who travel each morning in opposite directions, returning at sunset to recount the

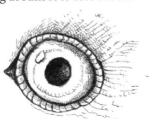

Honor Mother Earth and living things, guarding and honoring the divine magic that lives within you.

secrets of the world to the god. Like the unknown, mystery, and death, the Raven may scare us, because it harbors a darkness that we deny we have within us, projecting it outside. But it is precisely into that darkness that it invites us to enter, because only in darkness will we learn to become enlightened and take the step needed to stir our inner awakening. A step beyond the fear of darkness and shadows, recognizing them as part of us and for being able to discover the treasures they conceal.
The Raven teaches us to draw with respect, love, and humility on the pure potential of the creative source. To look into our depths and guide the energy flows within us. To discover the magic that lives within us and learn how to use it, showing us that we are all sorceresses and sorcerers.

AWARENESS QUESTIONS

~ Are you afraid of your personal magic?
~ Do you study it, explore it, or deny it?
~ Can you accept mystery as a divine gift, placing it at the service of your growth, or limit its power by trying to analyze it?
~ Do you honor the sorceress or sorcerer within you?
~ Do you use your energy to wish that evil or blessings may fall upon your neighbor?

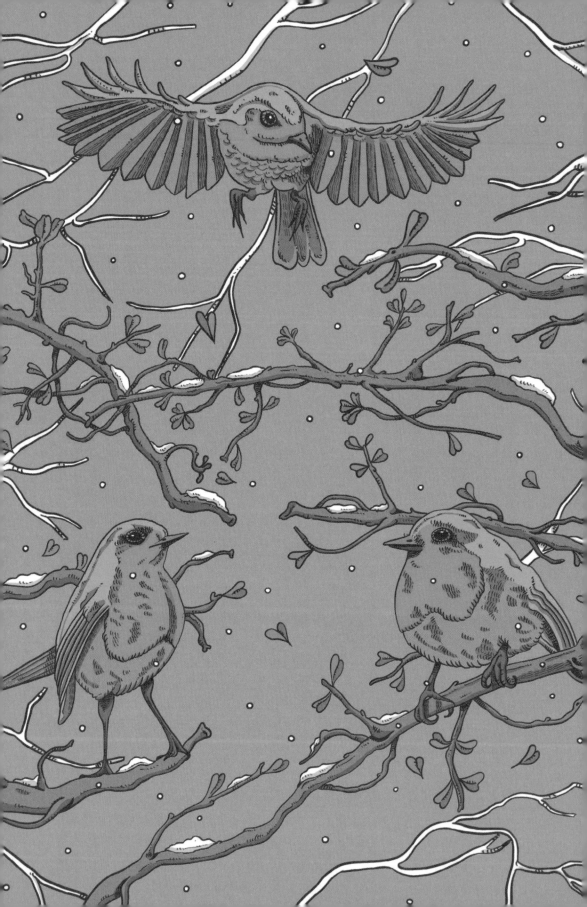

THE ROBIN
The Friend
Offering Comfort

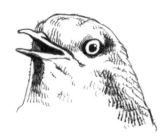

L ovable, endearing, and comical at the same time, the Robin reconnects us to the innocence of the inner child, to the relief that comes from being able to count on a greater force that will take care of us. This small bird generates hilarity and closeness, thanks to its soft shape and its melodious song, which in winter resonates through the air, bringing hope and optimism just when the bright colors of summer give way to gray and windy skies, which cloud our mood in melancholy. This small and combative bird arrives unexpectedly in front of our windows to bring us joy and levity stemming from sharing our experience spontaneously. It heralds transition from fall to winter, anticipating the magical return of snow and with its colorful chest uplifts the spirit, bringing warmth and confidence. The Robin is a symbol of luck, goodness, and compassion, but also of renewal and rebirth. According to one myth, on the first night of Christmas the beating of its little wings was able to keep the fire burning in the grotto of Bethlehem where the Holy Family was sheltering. In the morning, its gray plumage had turned red, as a reward for its tenacity and resolve. It is no coincidence that this feathered friend is associated with Christmas and its festive atmosphere of celebration, intimacy, and sharing. The Robin brings us the medicine of comfort, reminding us how important it is to give and receive it, and encouraging us to empathize with others. It helps us understand that compassionate acts are reciprocated with gifts of gratitude from Life.

Breathe when you see me. Your pleas have been heard.

AWARENESS QUESTIONS

~ Can you rejoice in Life simply because you exist?

~ If you see someone in trouble, are you moved by compassion, or do you remain indifferent?

~ Are you capable of comforting someone honestly? Do you let yourself be comforted?

~ Do you believe that when you close one cycle, you always open the next one?

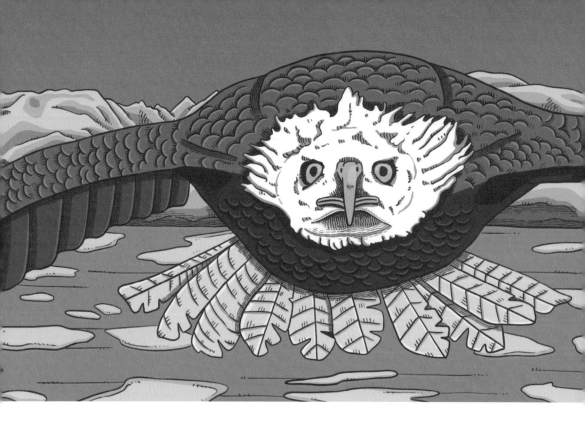

THE EAGLE
The Manifestation of the Spirit

From time immemorial, this bird of prey has been associated with spiritual power; in fact, the Eagle invites us to spread our wings to soar to the heights of the world and draw in the grandeur of the Spirit. It is one of the most coveted totem animals; it is the undisputed ruler of the heavens and represents the ability to remain connected to one's Spirit while living on Earth. It is a symbol of freedom, grace, openness, and expansion: all attributes achieved through a process of profound inner growth. The feathers of the Eagle have graced the heads of warriors and

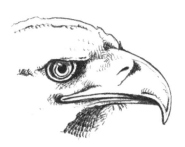

Extend your vision and you will see the magnificence of the universal design.

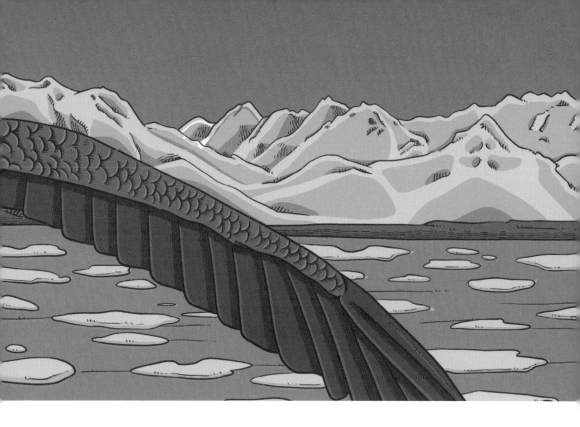

leaders; they have been, and still are, shamanic tools for energy healing and deep cleansing of the subtle bodies: i.e., the life force present within each of us. For Native Americans, the Eagles were a sign of the presence of the Great Spirit, therefore venerated and held in great esteem. They tell of heights to be reached in order to see clearly, to have a global and unitary vision of things. The Eagle nests in the high mountains, where the sky is clear and the air is crisp, showing us how important it is to breed and give birth to our projects in environments suitable for their development. How can new ideas come into the world unless the right environment is there for embracing them? In Greek mythology, the Eagle is associated with Zeus, who often transformed himself into an Eagle to appear to humans. Because of its ability to look into the sun, in the Christian religion this bird is associated with the resurrection and represents the Apostle John. The animals that symbolize the apostles are considered the strongest.

AWARENESS QUESTIONS

~ Do you recognize the Divine within you?
~ Are you connected to your Spiritual energy?
~ Is the space where you live suitable for developing new projects?
~ Can you accept your own Light and the Light of others?
~ Do you occasionally allow yourself to look at things from above, so you can broaden your comprehension?

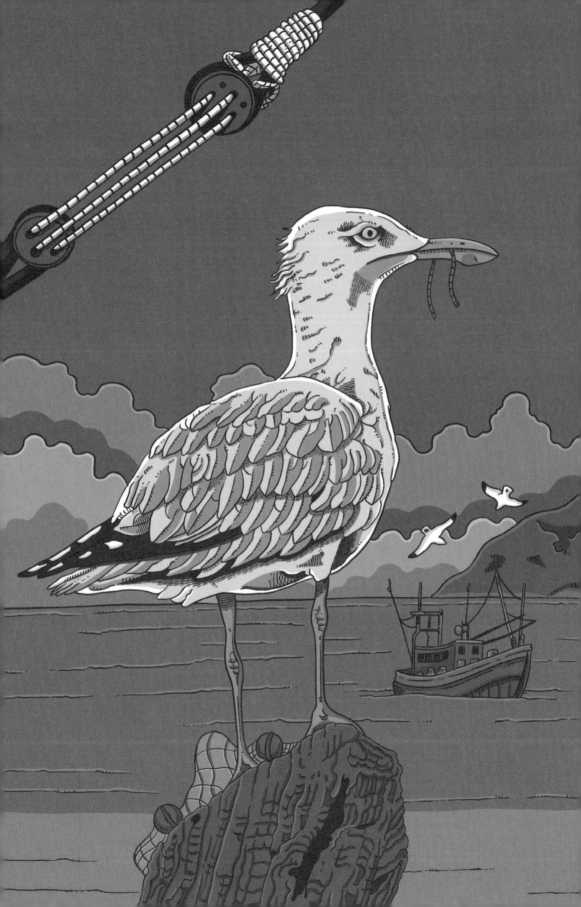

THE GULL
On the Wing
with a Light Heart

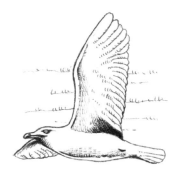

This big, shore-hopping bird is a master at adapting to city and inland living, in places crossed by a river or a waterway. It brings us the medicine of carefreeness. And it also explains how to reach this state. Its breezy, clumsy, and graceful flight shows us that by adapting to what Life throws at us and by not leting the bar of our aspirations and expectations get set too high, we can embrace the spirit of freedom that comes with being carefree. When fishing is tough, there will be a fishing boat to land on and feed; when the ocean is empty, there will be food others have discarded. The Gull shows us that a light-hearted attitude comes from the ability to adapt and be flexible, abandoning rigid thinking and beliefs that shape reality as if it were a one-way boulevard. The Gull invites you to be

Trust in Life.
Soar above boxed-in
 thinking and embrace
freedom.

open-minded, to seek out adventure and the unknown, fully believing you will find what you need.
Maybe it's not what you were hoping for, but it will be enough. Stay open-minded; being carefree is not the same as being indifferent or not caring.

AWARENESS QUESTIONS

~ Do you have space for carefree living in your Life,
   or do you think you need to keep everything in check?
~ Can you adapt to the unexpected?
~ Is your attitude toward Life trusting, or are you scared of losing control?

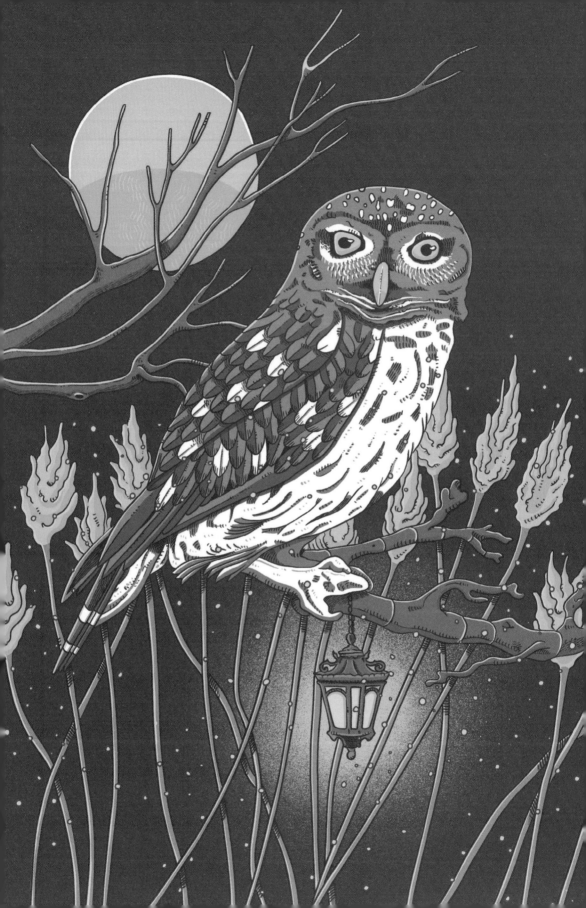

THE SMALL OWL
Razor-sharp Sight

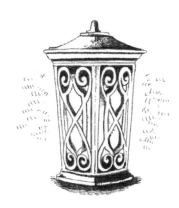

A lunar creature linked to the Great Mother, this bird embodies the indomitable and the wild, coupled with the ability to create and decompose. Its proximity to darkness and the night means the Small Owl is an animal with a dual meaning. With its gleaming gaze, it brings us the gift of wisdom and knowledge, possessed by those that have a deep understanding of the laws of the world and its creatures. Associated with death, this bird is often depicted in monumental cemeteries. For the Small Owl, even things shrouded in darkness are predictable and clear. It is not afraid of what is hidden and what is not shown but is there. Its wisdom is rational, the fruit of a sharp and attendant, attentive and mnemonic mind. In ancient Greece, this creature was attributed with glaukopis, or a "bright and sparkling gaze." The Small Owl was moreover sacred to Athena, goddess of strategy, philosophy, and wisdom. Because of this association, its scientific name is *Athene Noctua*.

It invites us to focus on the light concealed in the darkness, for seizing everything that is divine and supernatural. It urges us not to become entangled in the web of indecision that is the result of an inattentive and confused outlook.

Penetrate darkness and seize the light that you will find there.

AWARENESS QUESTIONS

~ Does darkness scare you and throw you off balance?
~ When your view of events is clouded, do you look for guidance in reason and use the sharpness of your mind?

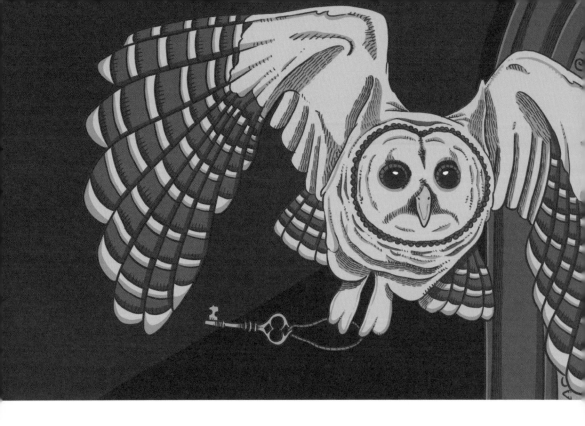

THE LARGE OWL
Intuition is Power

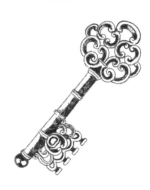

L ike the small owl, the Large Owl is one of the nocturnal animals by definition. Its ability to fly undetected has made it an ally of sorceresses and sorcerers. In fairy tales and in fantasy filmography, this bird is often represented as the wise helper and dispenser of advice. In popular religious tradition, with negative connotations, it was believed that the Owl's appearance could be assumed precisely by the familiars of sorceresses and sorcerers: that is, their allied spirits, considered minor and evil demons. So, this bird has a reputation for being a bad omen.

By day it is perfectly blended in with its surroundings, while by night it swoops silently through the dark, perceiving every sound. The Large Owl is always alert and aware. The medicine that it jealously guards and releases in our psyche, when we activate its force in us, is called intuition. With the Large

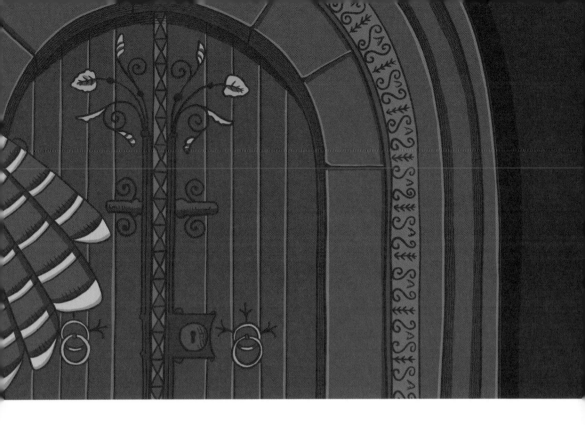

Owl flying across our inner skies, we do not need to investigate and seek confirmation, we just simply know. The truth stands certain and as clear as the light of day before our eyes. By perceiving it, we can see inside events and situations. Nothing and no one can deceive us.

If the Large Owl is your animal guide, it is your intuition that guides you. You only have to trust it and embrace its power.

I'm open to intuition and everything becomes clear to me. Faced with an infinite number of doors, I calmly choose the right one.

AWARENESS QUESTIONS

~ Do you trust your intuition?
   If the answer is no, what wounds of the Soul have not yet healed?
~ What relationship do you have with your innate ability to discover the truth inherent in events?
~ For you does the night—as a symbol of what is unknown—represent a threat, or a possibility?

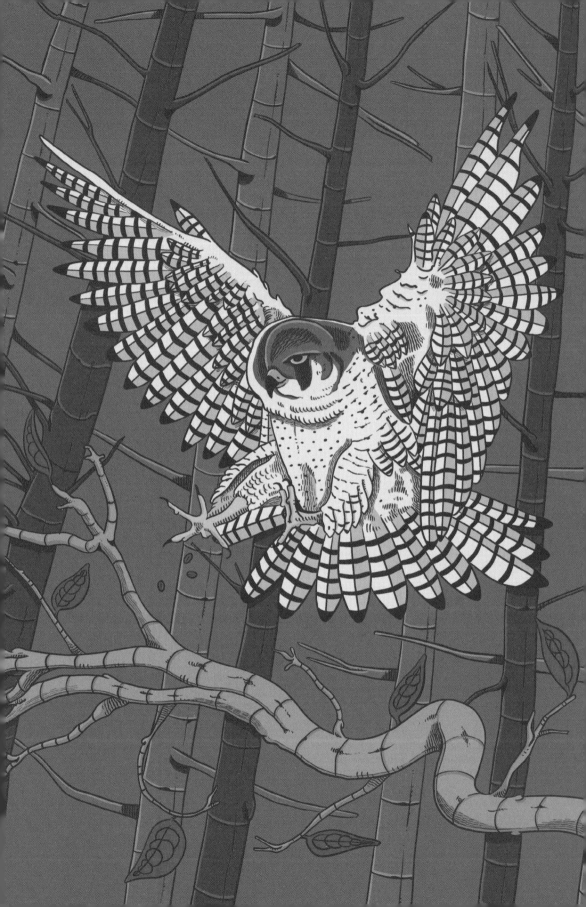

THE FALCON
Our Ancestors' Messenger

The Falcon speeds to deliver a message of reawakening and awareness at times when emotions get the upper hand, so much so that they push us off balance and distract us from living in the moment. This bird is the messenger sent by our ancestors, the wise roots anchoring our family tree, from which an enormous wealth of experience and knowledge stems. When we see the Falcon coming, we should stop, detach ourselves emotionally from the situations in which we are immersed, and listen to the advice that our ancestors bring us from the depths of the Earth and from the heights of the sidereal regions.

> Have you perhaps forgotten who you really are? Shout it out, so that you may experience a reawakening.

Earthly but also heavenly ancestors considered a traveler between the worlds, the Falcon, as a symbol of cosmic spiritual force, and as an attribute of many deities: Hermes, Horus, Apollo, Odin, Freya, and others. It is the Simurgh, the bird that spreads all the seeds of the Tree of Life on Earth; it is Gayatri, the bird that brings the Soma, the drink of immortality, into the world. In Ancient Egypt, the god Horus, who ruled every element and was associated with the creative power of the sun, was depicted with the head of a Falcon. It reminds us of the power and strength of our Spirit, reminding us that we do not need to beg for recognition and attention from others, but that we can affirm these stimuli within us, so that we can then manifest them to others. When you meet a Falcon, you should know that it is coming to encourage you to be honest and to fully appreciate yourself, your merits, and your worth.

AWARENESS QUESTIONS

~ What is gripping your attention to such an extent that it is causing you to lose contact with your reality?

~ Are you responding proactively and consciously to what Life is bringing you?

~ Are you honoring your ancestors' wisdom?

~ Do you let yourself listen to the wisdom of your Spirit?

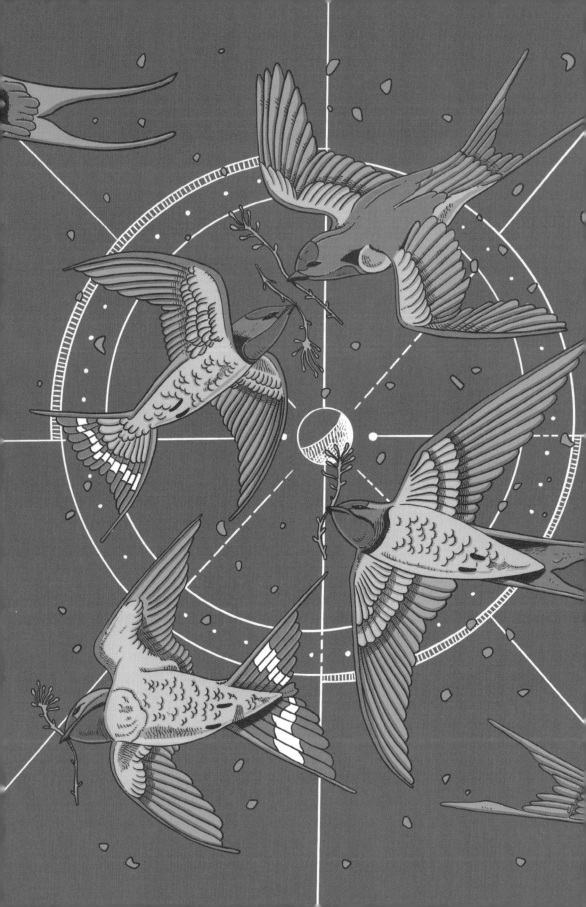

THE SWALLOW
The Lady of Rebirth

Agile, unconstrained, and defined by elegant black feathers, the Swallow announces the return of Spring, and it is strange that this bird should choose to do it dressed in black and not adorned with more colorful and flamboyant hues. Black bestows authority, power, and centering energy, and the Swallow is like an orchestra conductor who instructs nature to express all facets of its being, in every song and sound hailing birth and rebirth. This creature plays an important role, and the power it gives is the fruit of experience as a traveler, as a connoisseur of many places around the world. It is a lady of the threshold, but it does not guide us from light to darkness, but quite the opposite. From nest to the world, from the womb to Life. And its back is covered by a black cloak of feathers; its chest sports lighter hues, adorned with red and blue. When Swallows are spied in the sky, our Hearts open up, a smile lights up our face, and our expression is flushed with joy. The sun is warm again, gems burst into flowers, and the air is heavy with their scent, while cherry trees are tinged pink and the green of each leaf breathes new life. The Swallow returning from its migratory journey, along with the whole flock, is nature reawakening in a new cycle of birth and rebirth. For Christians, it symbolizes the resurrection of Christ at Easter, and according to an Armenian legend it was the Swallows who bore witness to the miracle that took place. They were also attributes of Isis and were chosen by the goddess to announce the return of Osiris from the afterlife. For sailors this bird symbolizes the mainland, therefore the hope of returning home. In particular, the English sailors used to get a swallow tattoo after crossing the equator.

> Everything that dies is then reborn. Internalize this knowledge, and you can let joy in.

AWARENESS QUESTIONS

~ Do you believe that spring will always follow winter?
~ When the environment around you becomes hostile to your well-being, do you allow yourself to migrate to more sunny and welcoming places for your Soul?
~ Do you share with your elective family the joy of each of your rebirths?

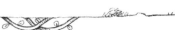

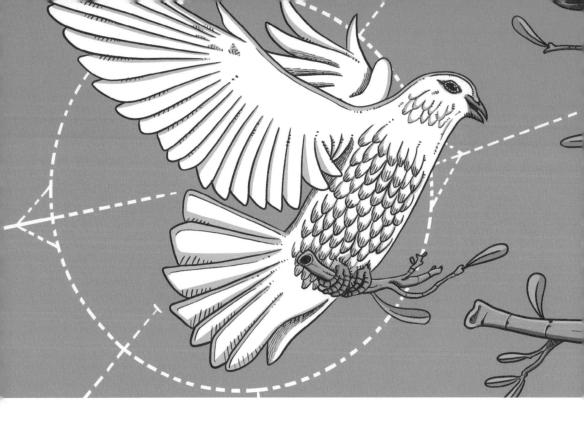

THE DOVE
The Priestess of Pace

L ike a priestess in the act of celebrating a ritual, in its white robe the Dove embodies purity, righteousness, integrity, and peace. In the Phoenician language this bird's name means "priestess" and many myths narrate that this divine animal is the bearer of the power to speak oracles, to channelize, and to prophesize. The Dove has been associated over the centuries with the Sibyls, with the goddess Venus, and with Mary Magdalene; it was also the only animal that could approach the Oracle of Delphi and, in the

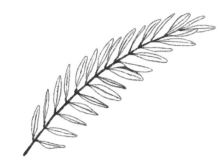

I entrust myself to the priestess who lives within me, and I ask her to guide me so that at all times I am aware of my divinity.

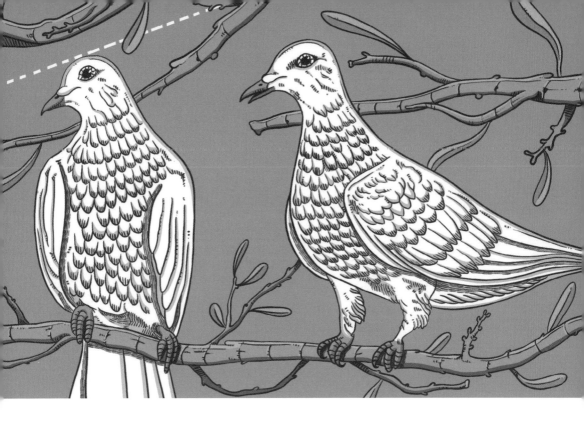

Christian religion, it was elevated to a symbol of the Holy Ghost. A white dove returned to Noah's Ark carrying an olive branch, confirming that the Earth had resurfaced from the water. It symbolizes the joy of the Spirit, faith, the heavenly love that is the forerunner of Peace, reminding us that we come from the divine. The Dove invites us to connect to our Heart, to its purity, to the innocence that inhabits it, urging us to awaken the Priestess or the Priest within us, to act with integrity and rectitude, fully in harmony with divine grace. This bird urges us to be a channel between heaven and earth, to unite these two realities within us, to meet peace throughout our Life on this Earth. The Dove invites us to listen and to speak the truth, which as incarnated souls we have been selected to bring to this planet.

AWARENESS QUESTIONS

~ Do you feel you are a channel of heaven and earth?
~ Are you in touch with your integrity, your innocence, your inner peace, which resist, regardless of the event?
~ Do you recognize yourself as a divine being?
~ Have you awakened the archetype of the priestess or the priest within you?

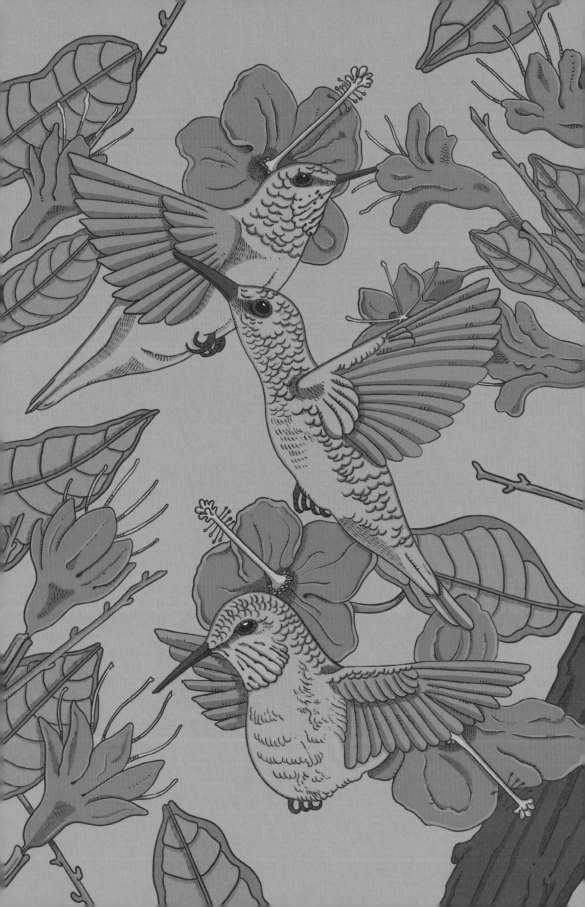

THE HUMMINGBIRD

Lust for Life

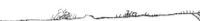

Tiny and with the ability to hover while also remaining immobile, the Hummingbird is here to show us how awesome it is to experience the joie de vivre, savoring the moment to the full. For this bird, there is no past, there is no future, but only the eternal present; and it is precisely this awareness that gives rise to and manifests his healing power. It feeds on flower nectar, the food with the highest vibrations after fruit, and this can only fuel and energize its joy of living. In fact, food impacts our mood, and the Hummingbird reveals this secret to us. It loves beauty, recognizing it, courting it, and bringing it into the world by spreading its vibrations. It invites us to open our hearts, to live our days with gratitude because they are a gift. Being here to live the human

> There is nothing more awesome than feeling alive and enjoying the gift of life.

experience is not a foregone conclusion. It is a gift; and if we recognize it as such, we have a duty to open ourselves to receive the wonder that characterizes each creation in the universe. The Hummingbird shows us the way to enjoy the divine abundance available in this earthly sphere and encourages us to honor the freedom inherent in our spiritual nature. If locked up in a cage, this creature will die immediately, demonstrating that even the lust for life will be extinguished when we feel imprisoned, restrained, and forced to do or be something that fails to resonate with our hearts.

AWARENESS QUESTIONS

~ How is your Heart doing? Is it free to sing about its truth?

~ Do you allow yourself to freely express the love you feel for yourself and others?

~ If your expression is not free, and does not flow, what is imprisoning you?

~ What is your relationship with beauty? Do you know how to embrace it? Do you allow yourself to create and share it?

~ What is your relationship with joy? Do you feel entitled to experience joy? Or when it emerges, do you feel guilty and so you reject it?

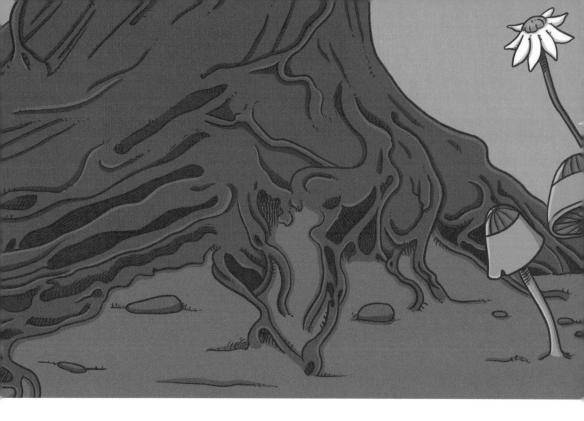

THE BLACKBIRD
The Skilled Communicator

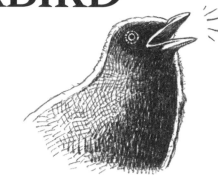

T he Blackbird is a skilled communicator. In fact, it uses its voice to sing melodious songs that fulfill various purposes and functions. It can be heard mainly at sunrise and sunset, as if opening and closing the day before the onset of night. Its harmonious songs mark these two moments of transit and have been celebrated by poets and lyricists. With its melodies, it reminds us that we can learn to combine words to talk about, ask, describe, praise, pray, create, and resolve conflicts. Communication can take place on many levels, but the Blackbird invites us to

Remember that you can use your voice to communicate who you are, revealing each and every nuance. Do not limit yourself to expressing a single facet of you.

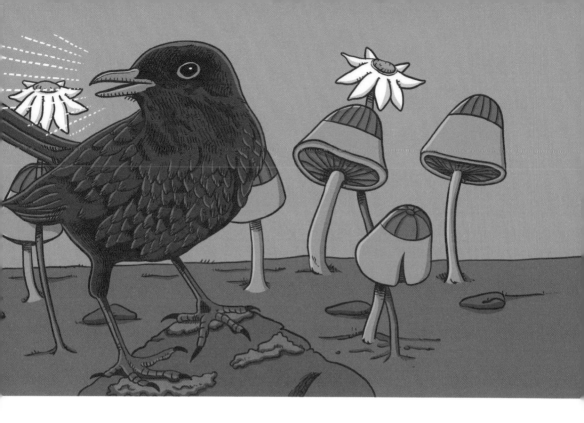

pay attention to verbal communication: a very powerful tool that we can use to create harmony or discord, both without and around us. This animal tells us that to be a skilled communicator, we need to be a good listener too. We need to listen to our emotions and needs, and obviously also to those of others. If we do not consciously listen to what is stirring our emotions, then how will we be able to communicate it? And if we do not do the same with others, then how will we be able to understand them? The Blackbird is associated with the figure of the thinker, the philosopher, the artist who expresses himself with his voice, with words; with creatives who are able to bring to light new aspects of reality, who do not limit themselves to reciting scripts that have already been written, but inventing new ones and also allowing themselves to embrace improvisation. By relying on the power of creation within us, communication becomes inspired, becoming a river flowing directly from the divine source. The Celtic peoples revere the three Blackbirds of the goddess Rhiannon, that from the branches of the Tree of Life exchanged messages between the realms of the living and the dead.

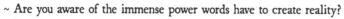

AWARENESS QUESTIONS

~ Are you aware of the immense power words have to create reality?
~ Do you communicate effectively?
~ Have you ever heard of empathetic or non-violent communication?

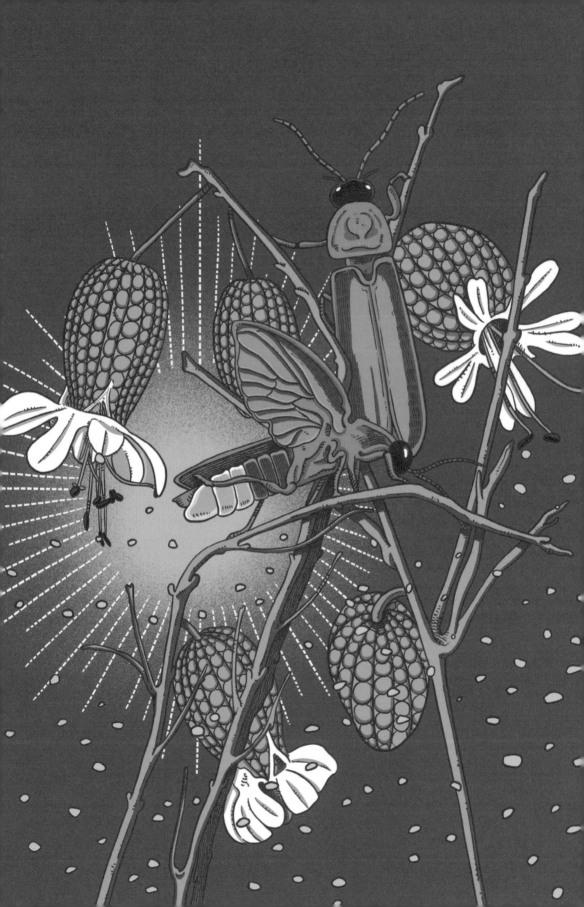

THE FIREFLY
The Light-emitting Creature

T he light of which the Firefly speaks to us is an inner light that always glows brightly, one that reveals our origin and is expressed in the act of giving oneself. These animals immediately reconnect us to the natural magic of the Earth, the world of fairies and the Little People in general. They take us back to a dreamlike, fairy-tale, otherworldly dimension, where—as in the typical magical vision of children—everything becomes possible and real. Who hasn't searched for them on hot summer evenings to awaken the magical part within us? Their bioluminescence comes from an oxidation process and

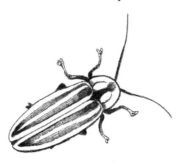

You can illuminate others without hiding in the darkness yourself.

is used both to attract their partner and to defend against predators. The Firefly therefore invites us to use our inner light to consciously choose who we want to surround ourselves with and who or what we want to attract to us. And at the same time, it encourages us to use it to discern clearly from whom we want to protect ourselves. This creature invites us to shine, but without splendor, without pomp, in a humble but non-dismissive way, always remaining connected to our inner magic, to the light-heartedness of the Spirit. In ancient Rome, Fireflies were considered carriers bringing balance and harmony, and they were the messengers of the goddess Diana, also called Lucina precisely because of her association with the Moon, of which she was a symbol.

AWARENESS QUESTIONS

~ Do you allow yourself to shine? Do you just let it happen or do you flaunt it as a wound that has gone unnoticed?

~ Or do you deny it, because you think you do not belong to the light or do not belong to the beings of light?

~ Are you connected to that dreamlike part within you that makes Life more lighthearted and more enjoyable?

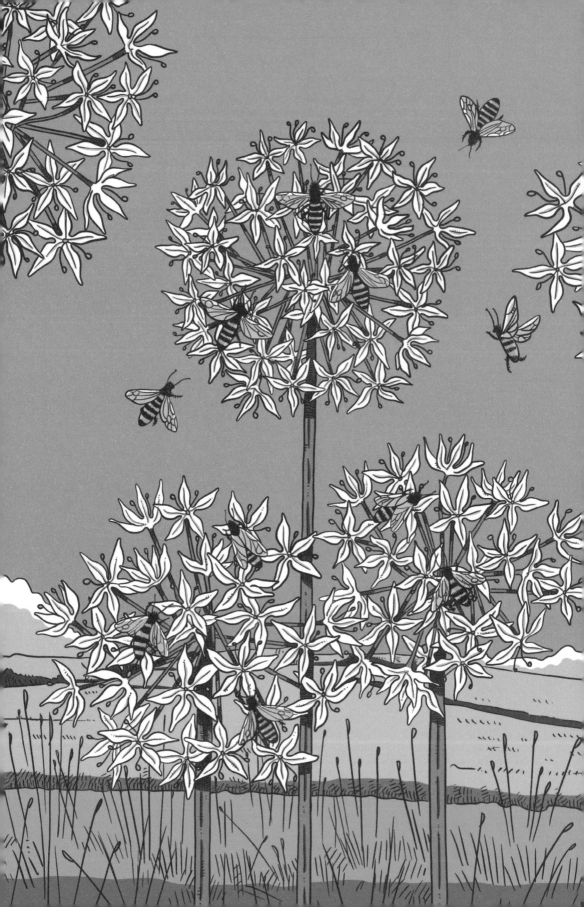

THE BEE
The Queen of Abundance

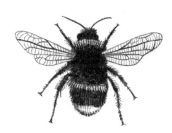

These flying creatures have been featured in mythology, in symbolism, in the arts, and in the cults of many peoples. Their way of life exemplifies a hierarchically structured society, a matrifocal community that functions perfectly. Each member of the hive responsibly accepts the power endowed by its role and expresses it, generating abundance and wealth at the service of the common good. The Bees embody the acceptance of their place in the world and thus contribute harmoniously to the advancement of Life. The Queen Bee is the attribute of the Great Mother, as the archetype of the fertile mother who generates all her daughters. Worker bees are a symbol of industriousness, diligence, care, wisdom, sweetness, and protection.

These animals invite us to co-operate, collaborate, and share, prioritizing the community and abandoning all forms of individualism. For the Ancient Egyptians, Bees were born from the tears of Ra and symbolized the Soul, purity, and the golden Sun pollinating the Earth, making it fertile with flowers and fruit. This role, together with the honey, royal jelly, propolis, and wax they produce, has always made them valuable: they provide food, medicines, and ritual tools, as well as precious gifts that man has made use of since Neolithic times, as shown by the frescoes on the walls of the cave of Altamira in Spain.

Commit to doing what you love, and abundance will be a flow running through you naturally.

AWARENESS QUESTIONS

~ Do you know how to enjoy the sweetness of Life?
~ Do you feel you are co-operating and working for the greater good through your actions?
~ Do you honor the mother who gave you Life?
~ Are you open to receiving abundance?

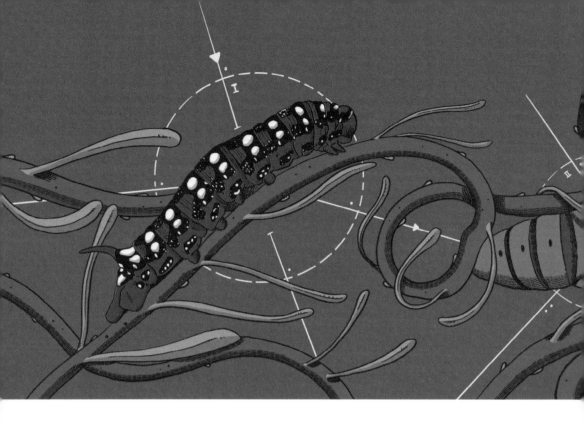

THE MOTH
The Power of Focus

Attracted by the Moon, the Moth moves through the darkness of the night, guided by a light that is more powerful, to confidently take the direction that appears marked out. It is a lunar animal, a night butterfly, a liminal being that marks times of passage, transitioning between one existential state to another. In urban surroundings, it follows the artificial light of the lamps and especially incandescent lamps, where it often encounters its demise. This creature therefore puts us on guard. We should not be dazzled by things that could become an obsession, causing us to

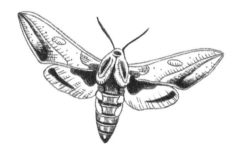

It brings clarity to your goals so you can pursue them tenaciously.

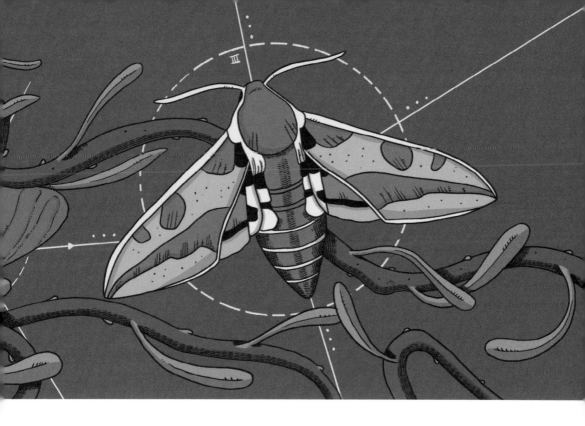

lose our critical and logical bearings. This creature invites us to tenaciously pursue our goals, remaining focused without losing contact with reality, our limits, our possibilities, and our resources. In this case, these goals, however ambitious, will become achievable for you. You will be guided so you can reach them. The Moth invites us to seek what enlightens us, spurring us to embark on spiritual research and undertake inner work,

to transmute everything that we have within us and everything that profoundly conditions our present state. This animal also shows us that in every event, you will be able to see and find the luminous part, the hidden teaching that, once revealed, becomes enchantment, magic, and amazement. It is associated with the spirits of the air, the dead, the beings who live on the other side of the veil and are present even if not visible.

AWARENESS QUESTIONS

~ What are your goals right now?
~ Do you feel focused on achievable goals or fantasies that have no chance of becoming reality?
~ When your direction is clear to you, are you able to follow it steadily, or do you constantly end up in dead ends that impede your progress?

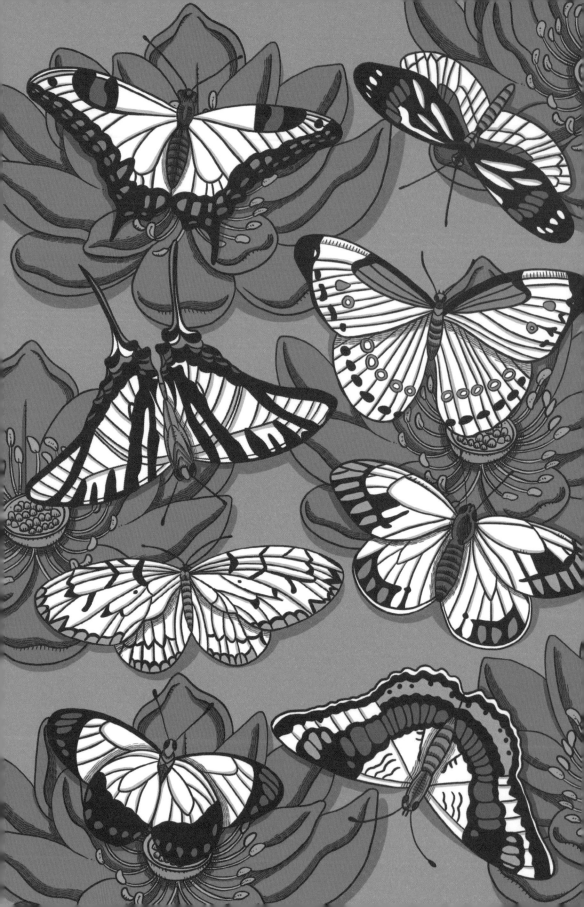

THE BUTTERFLY
The Transforming Dancer

The Butterfly is linked to the creative powers of the mind, to inspiration and to the world of ideas: when this animal crosses our path, we will experience an intuitive moment or have a new idea. White Butterflies are also messengers of the love emanated by guardian angels and angelic energies. They cause us to sense the closeness of loved ones that have passed, endowing us with a sense of grace and serenity. The different steps in the metamorphosis process are common to those of the creative process. The larval phase corresponds to its beginning: that is, to the moment of inspiration, in which ideas crowd the mind and it is not yet clear which direction they will take; the transformation into caterpillar coincides with the definition stage, when we choose what to do, even if we do not yet know how; the transition from caterpillar to chrysalis corresponds to the time of seclusion and self-listening, where the idea becomes a project. And, finally, metamorphosis into Butterfly represents the implementation of the

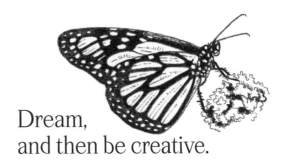

Dream, and then be creative.

project, when the thing we have created takes shape on Earth, and the Butterfly is ready to fly. Each of these steps requires dedication, care, faith, and acceptance, including the acceptance of possibly failing. If the caterpillar fails to accept the rhythm required for metamorphosis with humility, it will never turn into a Butterfly and will never experience the impalpable sense of freedom of lying in the air. This animal teaches us gracefully that the creative process consists of stages we need to pass through and times we need to respect to reach our goal.

AWARENESS QUESTIONS

~ At what stage of the creative process are you in with respect to your desires?
~ Are you open to new ideas?
~ What beliefs, habits, and family bonds are holding you back?
~ What do you need to change to enable you to take flight?

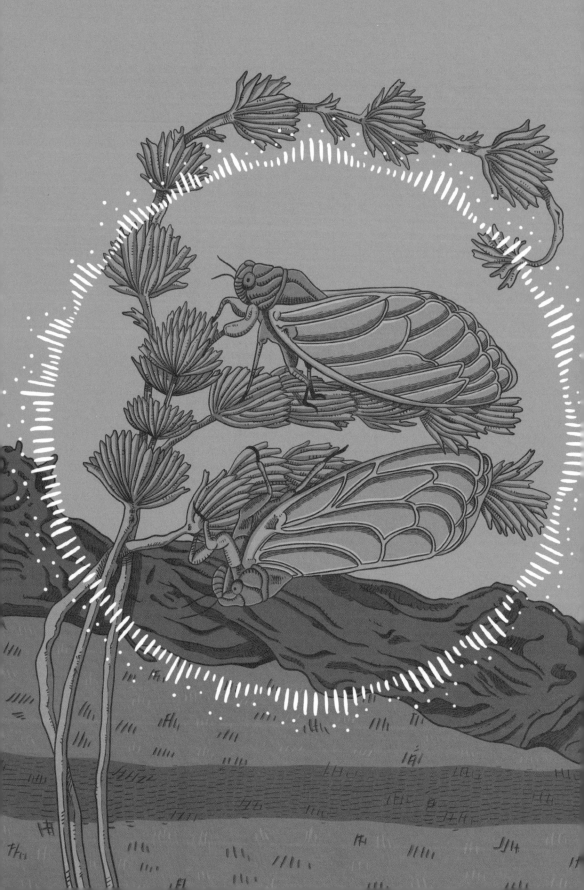

THE CICADA
The Hypnotic Musician

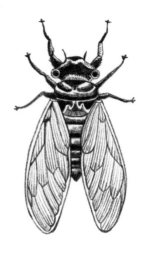

For Plato, Cicadas were men, so in love with the singing of the muses that they forgot to take care of their own basic needs. As a result, they expired and the Muses, created to celebrate music, turned them into Cicadas and sent them down on Earth to sing hypnotically and tirelessly. They are therefore a symbol of singing, of music, of ecstasy, but also of infatuation, of love that makes one lose all logic, and, just as under hypnosis, makes one subservient to the bewitching power of one's beloved. For me, they represent the summer, the warmth of the countryside and the parasol pine groves indigenous to Southern Italy, which is where I come from, and I've always liked the sound they make. I find it relaxing; it frees my mind from clutter and fleeting thoughts. Cicadas live as nymphs underground for several years, and then all together climb trees and complete their mutation, shedding their gold-colored outer husk, abandoning it on the bark. For a few months they live between the air and the earth. Males sing incessantly, emitting a mantra-like sound that attracts females. When they have laid their eggs on the bark of the trees and the nymphs have fallen to the ground, penetrating the earth, the adult insects will all die together, just as they had emerged into the light together. In Aesop's fables, Cicadas were seen as lazy, slouches that failed to care about vital needs, and so they were accused of not being prudent and realistic. This is a view that some people still have of artists. Art is considered a useless activity, when, instead, we know that it is pure nourishment for the Soul.

Find your unique voice and let it sing out.

AWARENESS QUESTIONS

~ Is your voice free to sing out whenever it feels the need?
~ What relationship do you have with singing and other forms of creative and artistic expression?
~ Do you allow yourself to fall in love and be so symbiotic with the other person that you overlook yourself?

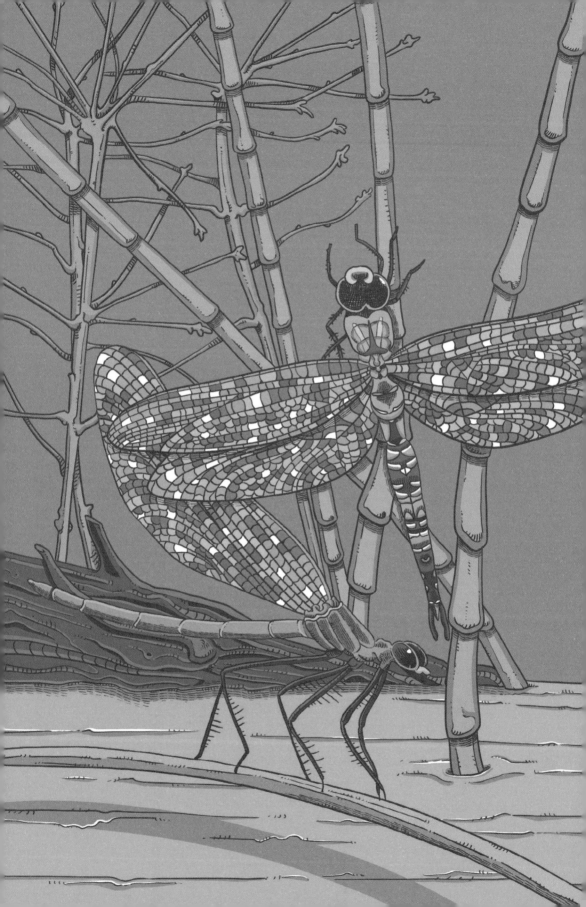

THE DRAGONFLY
The Clairvoyant

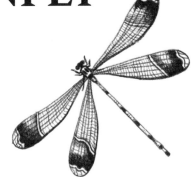

The Dragonfly proffers the power of a clear sight that guides us toward freedom and a state of emotional and physical balance. It encourages us to observe carefully, thanks to which we can take down the web of illusions and stories we tell ourselves. To dissolve these illusions, observing alone is not enough; we need to observe with awareness, by studying the dynamics and mechanisms that are acting within us, based on the rule that we see only what we can recognize. Illusions are the result of projections, desires, a pain linked to shortcomings; basically, they are a form of defense that prevents us from experiencing reality, savoring its intimate exquisiteness. This elegant insect has an extremely precise, 360-degree vision and, therefore, it is able to focus opportunely on the goals it wants to achieve. It is far-sighted, attentive, and determined, and this resolve is the result of knowing how to see clearly. The grace and agility of the Dragonfly is often associated

> Just walk away from illusions, leaving them to fall by the wayside, and let unconstrained freedom be revealed.

with fairies, who are depicted with the iridescent wings of this insect. It is a symbol of luck in many cultures, especially in Japan, but there are also negative features linked to the Dragonfly. In Europe, in times gone by, it was associated with witches and Satan and therefore disliked. And according to an ancient Native American legend, the Dragonfly was a magical dragon that, to deceive a coyote, turned into the insect we know today, continuing to inhabit its form.

AWARENESS QUESTIONS

~ Do you feel you have the power to see clearly?
~ Can you recognize and define illusions? Can you see the reality behind them?
~ Can you focus precisely on goals, when they become clear to you?

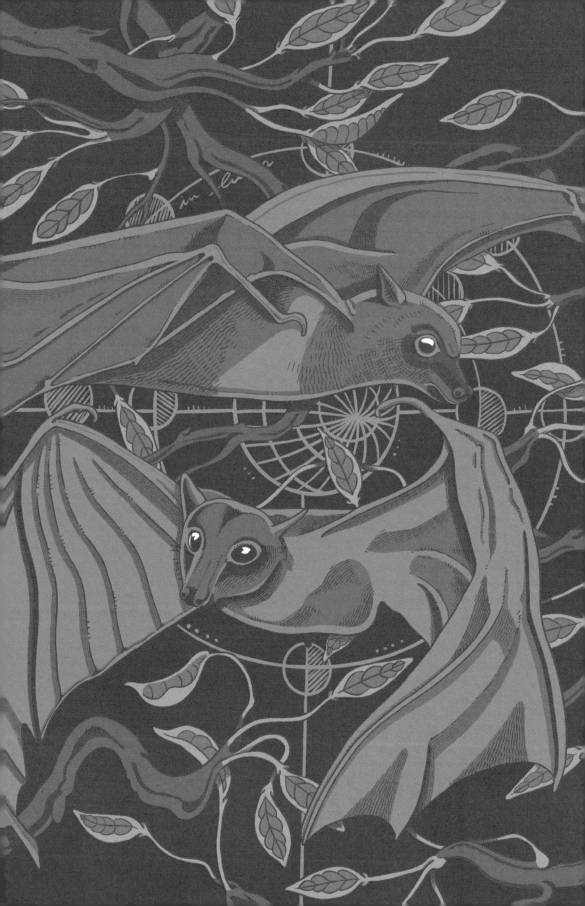

THE BAT
The Initiation Master of Ceremonies

I n figurative art, in literature and legends, its wings were the attribute of diabolical figures and vampires, and they were never lacking in witches' great cauldrons.

Bats have always been associated with the darkness they inhabit, with death, with the demonic. Bats are small mammals with wings formed by membranes and not feathers; they move in the dark using ultrasound and not sight. As a child, I was warned to be wary of Bats because they could get tangled in my hair. Now I know that was a superstition; but at the time, I believed

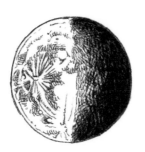

Come through fear, and it will become courage.

it: I still vividly remember the fear of walking in the evening on a street in my hometown, where they were always swirling around. As power animals, they invite us to overcome our fears by getting to know them. When a Bat flies in our inner night, in actual fact we are being called to descend into our fears and to examine them closely. Turning our viewpoint like it does, we will gain a new perspective which will give us confidence in our abilities. The Bat tells us about an initiation, crossing the Dark Night of the Soul, as Coelho calls it. And if there is a death that wants to reveal itself to us, then it is precisely an old part of us, marked by low self-esteem, distrust, and a sense of inadequacy. The sacrifice of the cowering victim enables the birth of the superhero. It is no coincidence that Batman has Bat wings.

AWARENESS QUESTIONS

~ Do you feel like the hero of your own life?
~ Do you believe that what scares you is an initiation that you need to go through?
~ How do you deal with your fears? Do you allow yourself to know them, so you understand where they come from? And do you feel they are real?
~ Have you already gone through initiations that have enabled you to grow?

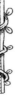

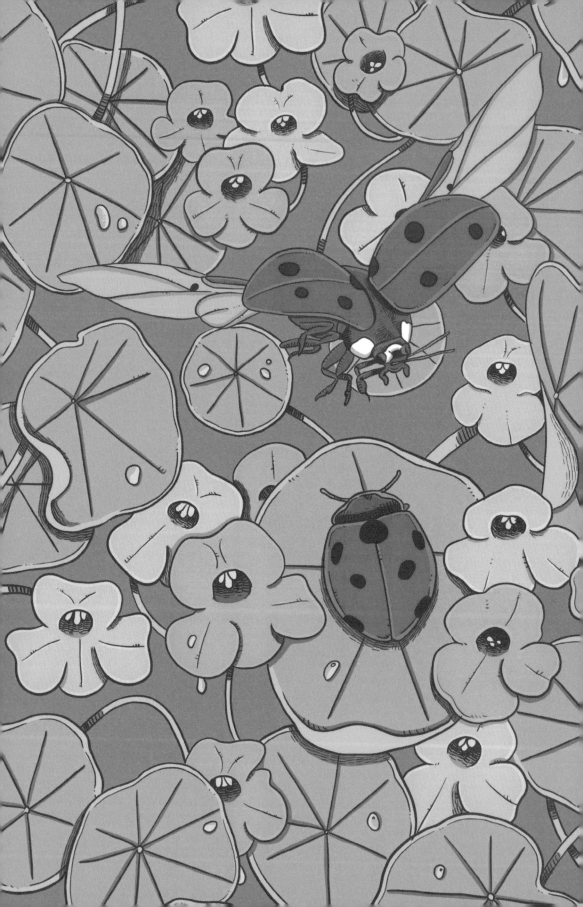

THE LADYBUG
The Dispenser of Fortune

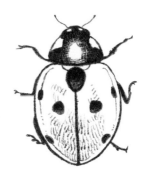

At every age and in every culture, the Ladybird has been considered a symbol of luck, prosperity, abundance, happiness, and good fortune. This attribution is probably due to the fact that Ladybugs feed on aphids, plant pests capable of destroying entire harvests. So, imagine in primarily peasant societies, such as those of the past, the value of the arrival of Ladybugs, seen as a sign of divine providence and good fortune. They are still used as a biological antagonist against plant parasites, precisely because they have a special appetite for them. This small beetle that owes its name to its scarlet color has therefore been one of man's great allies, inasmuch as it enabled man to grow his own food and feed himself. For this reason, it has been associated with many deities, including Freya, Hera, Lucina, the Virgin Mary, and Christ. According to a legend, the Ladybug was born from a drop of blood of a giant who lived in a world where death did not exist. It was the Ladybug that taught him the benefit of introducing it everywhere, so that all those who were worn out and tired could rest. This animal is the bearer of fairness, justice, and renewal. It invites us to draw on the life force and vigorous energy of our hearts, where every secret becomes visible and every solution is revealed. It tells us that within us, we have the key to solving any problem; we just need to be tuned in to the harmonious vibrations that beat within us, bringing renewal to our journey.

> Every problem has a solution, and the answer lies within; otherwise it would not exist. Let your Heart guide you to find it.

AWARENESS QUESTIONS

~ Do you think you're a lucky person?
~ Do you feel that cosmic forces are lending you a hand when you have problems?
~ Do you tend to look for solutions, or dwell on the problems?

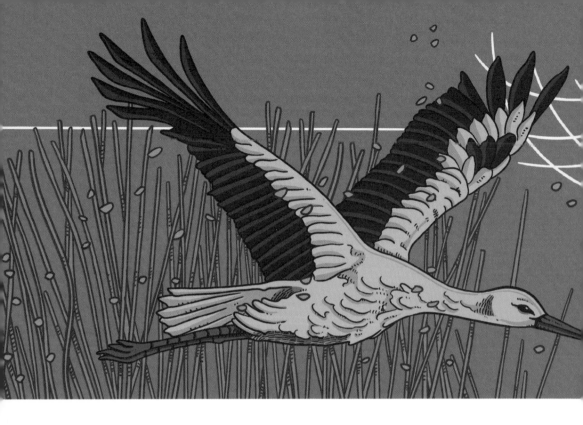

THE STORK
New Babies

Who as a child has not heard the story about Storks delivering babies? This legend has its origins in Eastern European countries, where, in spring, Storks migrated back from Africa and built their nests on chimney tops that were still smoking. Heated homes were primarily those with newborns, and this explains the correlation between babies and these animals. Their arrival in towns, however, marked nesting and then the arrival of baby Storks. The Stork invites us to embrace the new that Life offers us and to protect it until it is able to take wing by itself. It tells us that to let what is new in our Life, we need to create a nest suitable for its gestation; and it encourages us to be faithful to our wholeness, completeness, and integrity. This great migratory bird has been considered valuable since ancient times, seen as an attribute of the Great Mother and symbol of conjugal and filial love. The pairs of Storks are in fact faithful, and they diligently care for their offspring on top of the large nests they build. Offspring do the same when their parents become older, providing them with food that they would otherwise be unable to obtain. They were also appreciated for their ability to kill serpents; the Thessalonians, in Ancient Greece, held that killing a Stork was a crime.

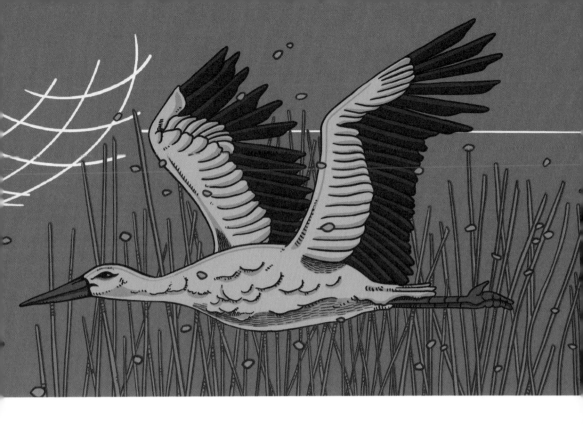

Whether you are
expecting it or not,
the new is on its way
and brings new balancing,
new views,
and new ways of taking
care of ourselves.

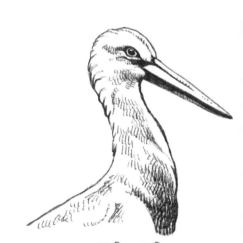

AWARENESS QUESTIONS

~ What would you like to renew in your Life?
~ For you, are new things a source of stress, or adventures to be experienced?
~ What are you willing to abandon to embrace what is new?

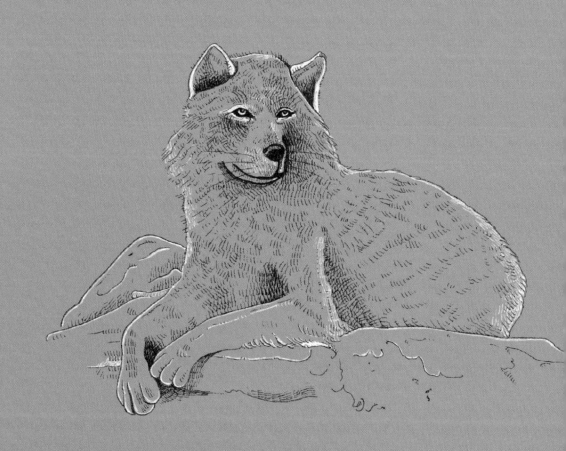

EARTH ELEMENT ANIMALS

Earth Element Animals present various characteristics in common with humans. Their medicines invite us to feel at one with our body, to use it in the best way as a precious tool, to honor it as a temple, and to inhabit it knowingly. They remind us to take root, to anchor ourselves to the Earth, and to explore it as a territory of our own being, as a home, as a mother. They speak to us of attributes, gifts, and teachings that we can experience, thanks to our animal, earthly, physical, and material parts of our being.

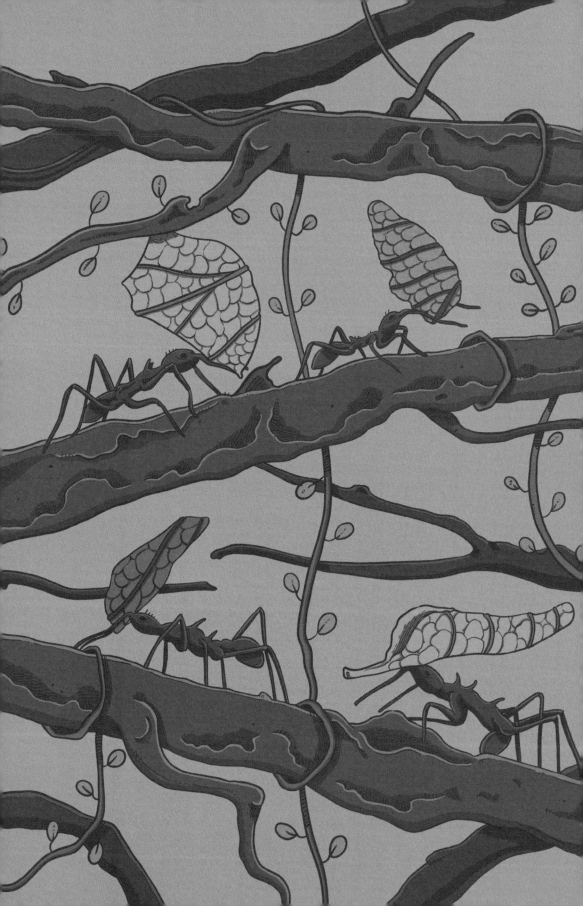

THE ANT
The Gatherer of Patience

Associated with willpower, determination, and perseverance, this small and robust insect reveals one of the key factors in the pursuit of our goals, as well as in overcoming obstacles: patience. In a society that propels us to seek pleasure in easy and immediate gratification, we desperately need this medicine. Like bees, Ants live in hierarchical societies and cooperate for the well-being of the community, to achieve common goals. In fact, they teach us the importance of teamwork, mutual help, co-operation, and, above all, organization. Ants leave nothing to chance, but program, manage, and rely on Mother Nature. Through this act of trust they practice the art of patience, endurance, and perseverance, especially when they make great efforts such as transporting food for the winter to the anthill. In Greek mythology, they were considered daughters of Mars, the god of war, and symbolized strength and determination. In actual fact, they live all over the planet, they adapt to all climatic conditions, and they can lift weights fifty times greater than that of their own body. Understanding the overlooked aspect of this archetype, we can note that if we totally identify with the rules of the group to which we belong, we may end up becoming rigid and inflexible, and this will surely lead us to sacrifice our individuality and personal well-being, as well as our capacity for self-fulfillment. Certain ants are also very aggressive; and, as we know, aggression at times can be a valuable tool for defending our borders. However, if we are constantly feeling angry, this may conceal pain for an unresolved issue.

Every little step
you take,
build your path.
Be patient and you
will see it be completed.

AWARENESS QUESTIONS

~ Walking the path to your goals, do you persevere, and are you organized and determined?

~ Is patience an attribute that accompanies you? Or do you want to obtain everything right away?

~ Do you allow yourself sufficient time to walk the paths you choose?

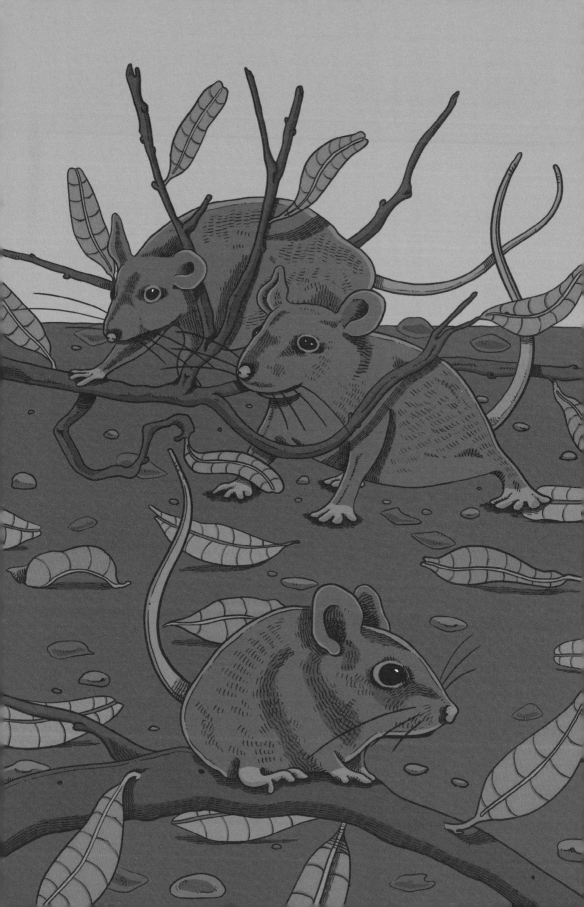

THE MOUSE
The Accuracy Specialist

crupulous, meticulous, thorough, and fussy: the Mouse does not let any detail slip through its fingers, and this allows it to observe the world around it and to notice things that inattentive people usually miss. Its medicine can help us focus on the substantial and deep meaning of a teaching we are learning; if we use it uninterruptedly, however, we risk caging ourselves in limiting patterns when we need broader horizons. The mouse is, indeed, a specialist, a creature which has devoted years of study and experience to a single field. It speaks to us, in fact, precisely about specialization of knowledge and tasks. Mice live within more or less large colonies, in which each mouse has its own role and well-defined tasks. They form pairs that can last a lifetime, and in serene environments they thrive and proliferate.

> If you get any closer and look carefully at every little detail, knowledge you cannot even imagine will be revealed to you.

Like us, they are sociable; they love to explore, play, and learn, and they need large spaces in which to live. Like us, if held in captivity or burdened with responsibilities that are too heavy to bear, they become stressed, compromising their health and well-being. Their genetics are very similar to ours, and we owe many of the advances made in human health to them. Mice cleanse mental energy of everything no longer needed, and they often use and validate what, for others, has now lost its function. This is why they are considered dirty and dangerous, as well as carriers of disease.

AWARENESS QUESTIONS

~ Can you dwell on what is important, to explore every little detail?

~ Do you consider yourself fussy, accurate? Are you far too much so that you are in danger of getting stuck, or is it a quality that you lack altogether?

~ When you are in nature, do you like to observe details, letting yourself be enchanted by the beauty of the microcosm, or do you prefer overall looks?

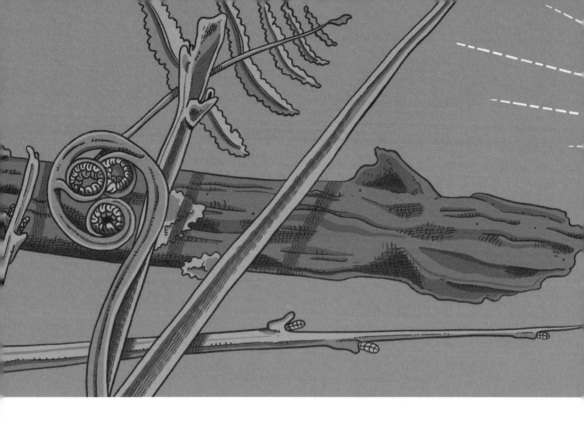

THE CRICKET
The Spirit Guide

Everyone is assigned at least one Spirit Guide. Let the voice of the Heart speak, and you will meet your own.

I f during the day the summer heat is celebrated by the song of the cicadas, at night it is praised by that of the Crickets. And it is precisely through their chirping, according to ancient legends, that it is possible to get in touch with one's spirit guide, namely with a wise force, inherent in oneself but identified in an external image, that helps people find their true nature and understand their true purposes in Life. The song of the Cricket, which

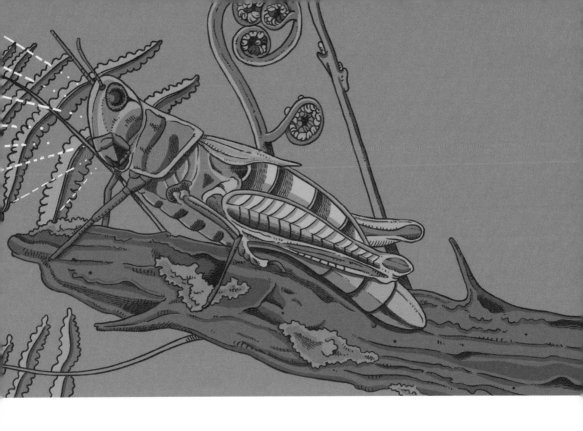

can be heard at considerable distances, creates harmonious vibrations that can dispel cumbersome thoughts and open a space for listening to one's inner voice, to receive the wisdom of one's spirit guide. It is depicted as such in many tales: for example, in Greek mythology it led Tiresias to the temple of Apollo, helping him to understand that its purpose is divination. In Ancient Egypt it accompanied the deceased to the afterlife, warning them of the dangers they might encounter on the journey. We also find it as a friend, adviser, and guide in the fantasy novel *Pinocchio*, where it helps the little puppet make the right decisions, warning him of dangers. Its role will be crucial for Pinocchio to become a responsible and mature human. The Cricket encourages awakening, awareness, rootedness, attention, and care for oneself and the purposes of one's Soul.

AWARENESS QUESTIONS

~ Are you in connection with your Spirit Guide?
~ Do you let those who are wiser help you, or do you think you have to do everything yourself?
~ Is the invisible world real, or fantasy, for you?

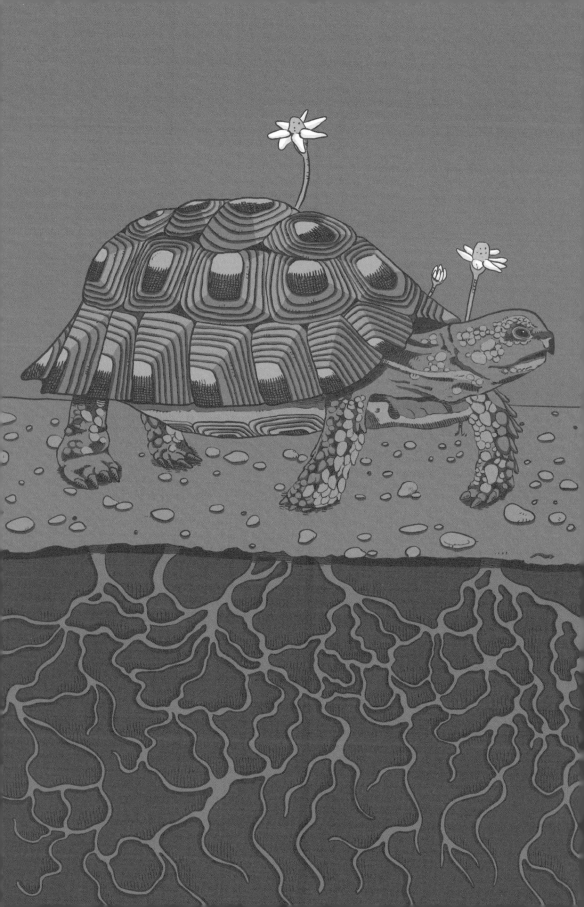

THE TURTLE
Mother Earth

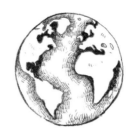

As ancient as our planet, long-lived, wise, resilient, fruitful, and inhabitant of both water and earth, the Turtle symbolizes the Great Mother, the begetter of all creatures. In shamanism around the world, it represents connection to the Earth—both as planet and element—rootedness, and the underworlds. In order to create deep trance states that made it possible, through sound, to connect with the Earth and elemental spirits, its carapace has been used by shamans in North America and Mongolia, as well as by the Tungusi and Han peoples of Asia and Australia to build solid, sturdy drums, believed to be sacred objects filled with Spirit. Its shell is a constant and efficient protection that it always carries, a home that contains it and provides extra protection from predators. It reminds us that we are children of the Earth, that it is to this Great Mother that we must turn when we need support and help. The Turtle/Mother tells us that we too, like all other animals, are her children and need to be humble in her presence, learning to receive with gratitude without taking on responsibilities of others, misunderstanding our role. By honoring the role of children, the Earth will give us everything we need: help, protection, support, nourishment, care, healing, regeneration, wisdom, and validation. The Turtle invites us to be rooted and fluid at the same time, living our present time creatively. It urges us to let our ideas develop before implementing them and to let go of those that do not have the necessary conditions to manifest solidly and strongly in the physical world.

> The child who remembers having a mother is never alone. The Earth is your Great Mother.

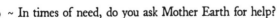

AWARENESS QUESTIONS

~ In times of need, do you ask Mother Earth for help?
~ Do you feel like her son/daughter?
~ Do you know how to slow down when it's time to do so, or does your haste prevent you from doing so?
~ What can you do to feel rooted, connected to nature, to the body?
~ Do you feel protected?

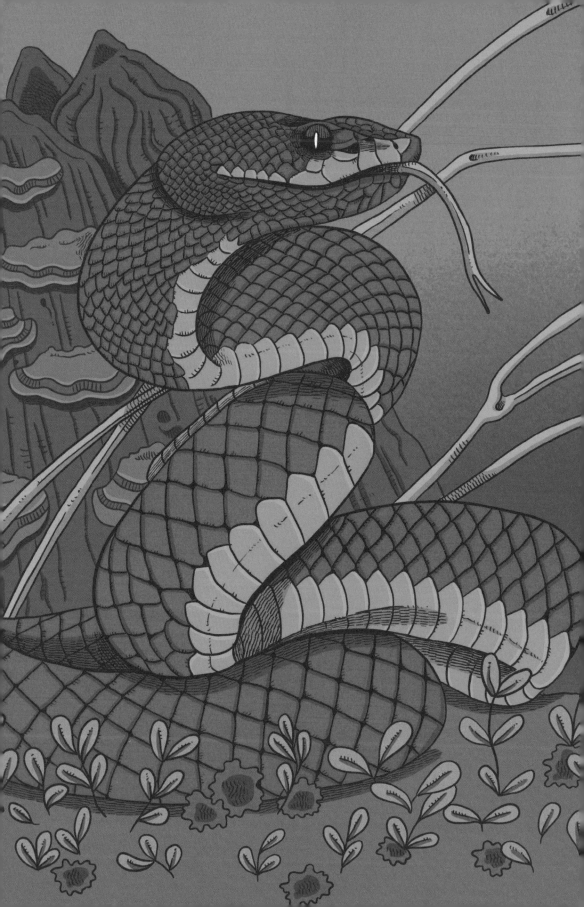

THE SNAKE
The Ever-changing Creature

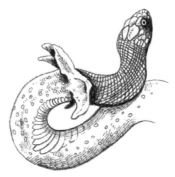

Powerful, chthonic, and ancestral, it slithers into the depths of the whole world; in some cultures it is revered, while in others it is demonized, but often it emerges as a deity, an ever-changing creature. It is able to let go of an unnecessary burden like no other, to transform and regenerate constantly, becoming a new Life form. In ancient cults of the Goddess, the Serpent is the wise guardian of sacred fire and of creative sexual energy, is the favored inhabitant of the Great Mother's womb, and accompanies initiates in the alchemical cycles of life-death-rebirth. The Serpent embodies the medicine of change, of knowing how to harmoniously blend with the waves of

> Change your skin as often as you feel it is tight, inappropriate, and worn out: the fire of regeneration will always burn in you.

Life in order to follow any possible future path, in full acceptance of all experience, without offering any resistance. It teaches us that suffering is rooted precisely in resistance to the flow of Life, and invites us to transmute emotional, mental, spiritual, and physical poisons through the powerful energy of change. It proffers the power of alchemical and transmutative fire. In Christianity and Judaism, it has been associated with temptation and the fall of man, and this has made it a nefarious symbol, around which a colorful range of legends has proliferated, arising to warn of the danger it represented. It is an initiatory animal that marks the often-fearful and therefore hindered passage from ignorance to knowledge, and therein lies the dark and negative interpretation of it.

AWARENESS QUESTIONS

~ What thoughts, actions, and desires do you need to transmute and be reborn?
~ Are there poisons in you that you want to turn into medicine?
~ Does changing your skin excite you or scare you?

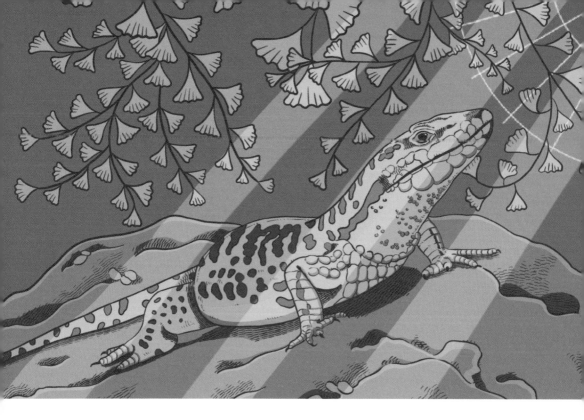

THE LIZARD
The Dreamer

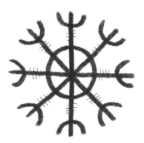

A s the sun warms it, it dreams and generates worlds that do not yet exist but can be created/built up by those who through imagination attract them, begin to desire them, and act to manifest them. The Lizard is a skilled dreamer and comes to show us that we inhabit multiple realities simultaneously. The dream world can be experienced consciously, lucidly, as shamans have always done. Through dreams, they perform healings, acquire new knowledge, perceive the world in depth, create, and communicate with spirits and ancestors. An attribute of the goddess Gaia, namely the Earth,

The creative process can only begin with dreams. So don't stop dreaming: otherwise, how can you shape your own reality?

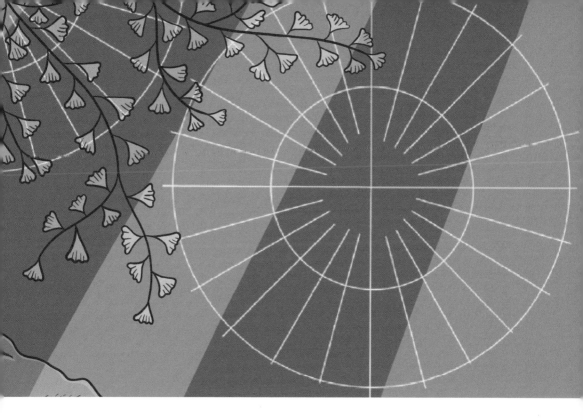

the Lizard was considered sacred and auspicious because, thanks to its ability to consciously live the Dream, it was able to know and predict the future, protecting those who were emotionally attached to it. It invites us to devote the right amount of time and attach importance to the dream world and thus to rest, to sleep, to that stillness of the body allowing us to delve into our imagination and explore other planes of existence. If attacked by predators, the Lizard sacrifices its tail to save its Life. In fact, it is able to get rid of it so as to distract the animal that is hunting it so it can flee. It will grow a new tail, less complex than the first one but still functional. This indicates that dreaming requires energy, courage, shrewdness, and a Spirit of Sacrifice: to make our dreams come true, we must be willing to let go of some parts of ourselves, believing that other—more essential—ones will grow in their place.

AWARENESS QUESTIONS

~ What are your dreams?

~ Which of them do you want to make come true?

~ What are you willing to sacrifice of yourself for this to happen?

~ Do you feel that you are living up to your dreams? If you don't, what makes you think you are not capable of realizing them?

~ Do you know that you are the Dream Come True of those who came before you?

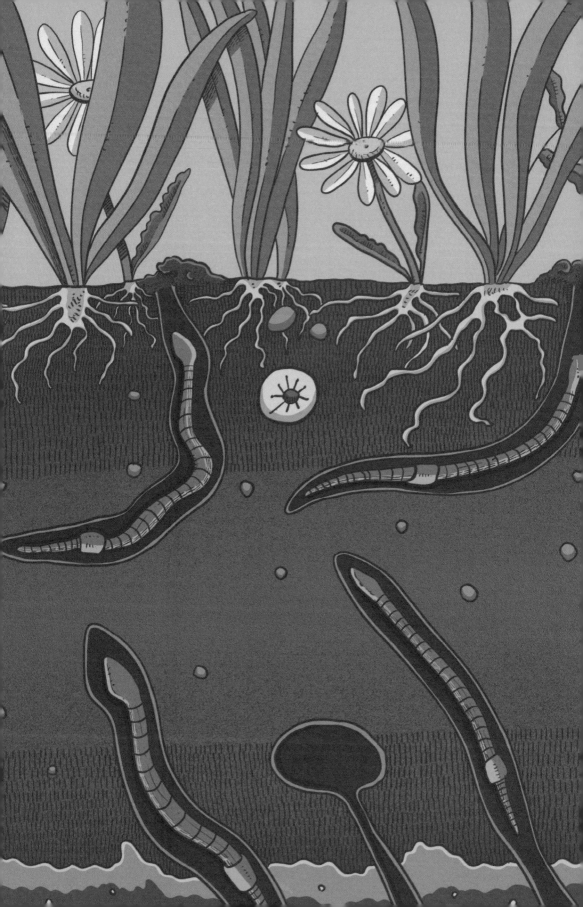

THE EARTHWORM

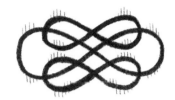

The Ability to Regenerate

One of the most fascinating and incredible beings of the subsoil is the Earthworm, tireless devourer of all rotting organic matter. It performs the magic of transforming leaves, grass, and all plant tissues which are destined to die into humus: a nutrient-rich soil that fertilizes the earth, making it suitable for hosting and supporting plant growth. It works this miracle simply by eating and expelling the products of digestion; and through this process it shows us how it is possible to regenerate and turn everything that has now lost its energy, its purpose, its meaning, into something new, useful, and vital. We too can internalize and digest our experiences, thus giving new meaning

to our days, transforming objects, homes, habits, and patterns. We can transform everything that is in our actual possession. The regeneration performed by this inhabitant of the dark womb of the Earth does not only take place in the soil, but also in the earthworm itself. In fact, in case of amputation, it is able to completely recreate the body segment containing the head, letting the missing part grow back just as the Lizard does its tail. According to other legends, it is able to split and regenerate both segments instead, creating from them two autonomous and independent individuals. The Earthworm lives underground and only comes out to eat, usually at night, or during periods of heavy rain so as not to drown. This humble invertebrate shows us that by operating silently, in our small way, we can go through great transmutations, revolutionary acts from which all Life can benefit.

> Anything that is doomed to die can become the fertile ground for rebirth.

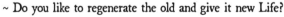

AWARENESS QUESTIONS

~ Do you like to regenerate the old and give it new Life?
~ Did you know that transforming oneself or unused objects is a revolutionary act?
~ Have you already experienced deep regenerations of your being? How do you feel after completing the process?

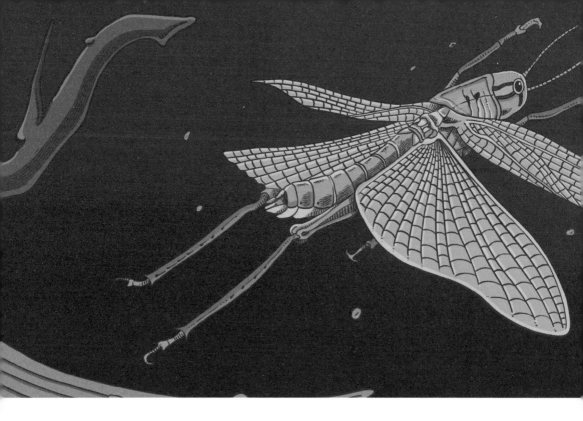

THE GRASSHOPPER
The Evolutionary Leap

I f we need to be spurred on to take that long-awaited leap, we can count on the Grasshopper, a professional jumper which is deeply faithful to its instincts and pace, ready to take a new direction freely and safely, toward new opportunities. A pioneer of new evolutionary paths, it opens dimensional doors and teaches us that, after great feats and bold leaps, there comes a time for rest, to recharge, to enjoy the newly conquered space and prepare for another leap. It tells us about faith, courage, and renewal, but also invites us to properly prepare

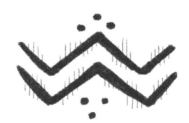

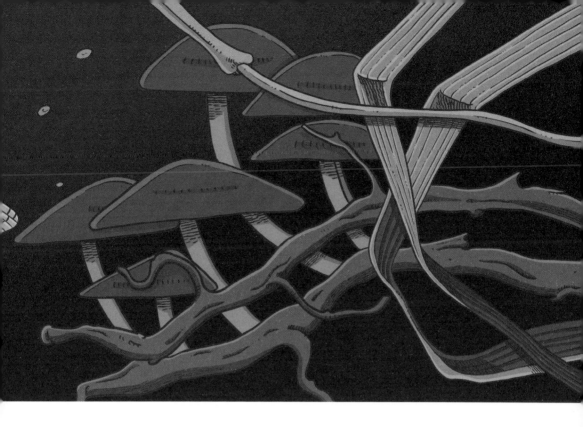

ourselves to gain the stability needed to sustain each evolutionary leap we take. There are changes that are made in small steps, while others require real leaps, acts of faith toward what we do not yet know but resonates deeply with us. Its color is green: present in nature in an infinite range of hues, it is also the color of our Heart chakra, which loves to renew itself, discover new things, and fearlessly dance free, celebrating what makes it feel alive and fulfilled.

Sometimes you just have to jump, leaving everything behind and trusting your own resources and qualities.

AWARENESS QUESTIONS

~ When your instincts keep telling you to take the leap, do you allow yourself to explore new opportunities?

~ Do you make progress in small steps, or do you like to take big leaps forward and seize opportunities that ensure great success?

~ Do you feel that the medicine of the Grasshopper belongs to you?

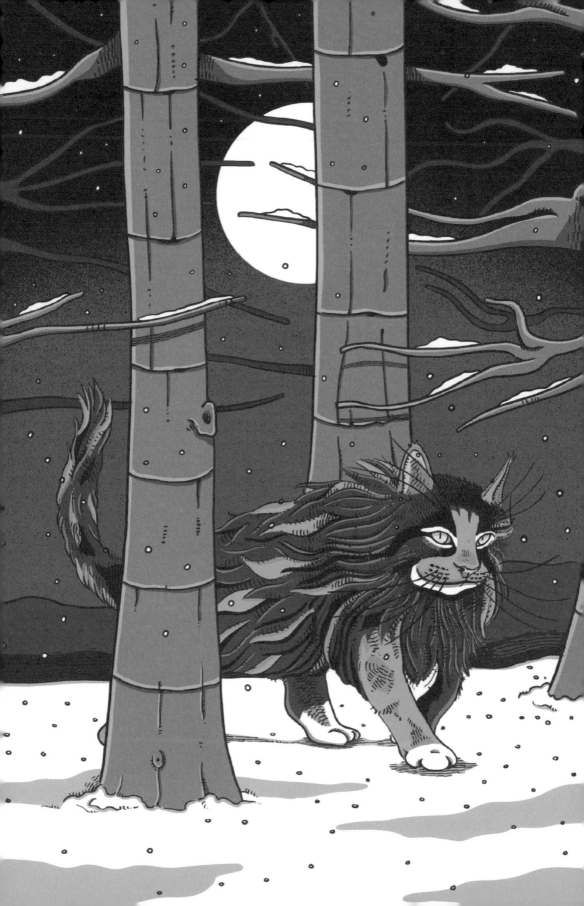

THE CAT
The Sacred Instinct

Mysterious, elusive, and only superficially tame, the Cat is the quintessential lunar and feminine animal. Despite being affectionate, sociable, and caring with humans, it is also very independent, showing a sinuosity and elegance typical of felines; it communicates eloquently through its body and does not allow its boundaries to be crossed, its instincts to be stifled, or its nature to be repressed. Linked to the world of spirits and energies, Cats are said to be the eyes of the gods, silently observing the dynamics of the world. In Ancient Egypt they were considered sacred as the personification of the goddess Bastet, she who could peer into the human soul and protect the home. The Cat's instinctive nature is not anarchy, selfishness, indifference, or distance; it is rather protection,

> My instinct is sacred, and I let myself be guided by it alone. I can let myself be tamed, but I do not forget my nature.

individualism, detachment, self-sufficiency, and compliance with the laws of nature that govern its role in creation. Like the Moon, it is also gentle and maternal; it can take care of itself and others; and its purr is an antidote to any sadness, sense of inadequacy, or emptiness: it is a healing animal. Not surprisingly, it is much loved and was already domesticated in ancient times for its ability to prey on rodents and insects that could create discomfort within domestic settings. It is believed to have the ability to protect homes from nefarious spirits. The Cat invites us not to give up the softness of affections and comforts, but to enjoy them to the full, always staying true to our innate power, which is sacred and reminds us of our true nature.

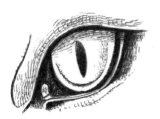

AWARENESS QUESTIONS

~ What is your relationship with your instinct? Do you know your wildness?
~ Do you welcome your lunar aspects? Can you take advantage of them?
~ Do you know how to recognize predators, those who want to make you reject your true nature?

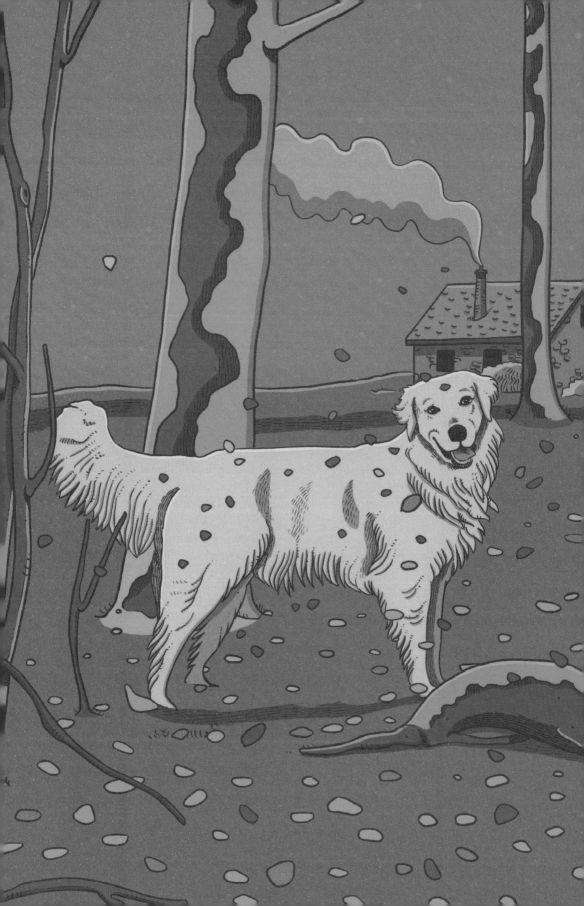

THE DOG
The Loyal Comrade

From time immemorial, dogs have been domesticated to protect human property, and to provide companionship, help, and comfort. They are loyal wolves who have chosen to put themselves at the service of a humanity that often abuses their helpfulness and kindness, denaturing them. Despite this, Dogs remain loyal to their mission and continue to show compassion for our limitations. In many mythological systems, Dogs are guardians of treasures, places, and precious goods: think of Anubis, Cerberus, Garmr, Orthrus, and Xolotl, just to name a few. Obviously, when we entrust a very valuable asset to someone, this someone must be trustworthy. Dogs, with their special

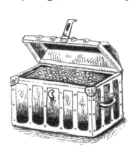

> The gift of loyal friends is a divine blessing that makes your Heart spread its wings. Acknowledge its value.

medicine, have always inspired trust in human beings. They are a symbol of loyalty to both their master and their pack, of protection of places and people, as well as of wisdom and friendship. I grew up with Dogs from an early age, and their friendly, playful, affectionate, and protective presence has been fundamental to my emotional development. I have always considered them friends, family members, beloved inhabitants of my Heart. The Dog teaches us to humbly put ourselves at the service of others, respecting the vision of our Soul, and invites us to be loyal to ourselves first, so that we in turn can be loyal to those surrounding us.

AWARENESS QUESTIONS

~ Do you consider yourself a loyal person?
~ Do you think that sometimes you are faithful just because you seek the approval of others?
~ If you feel the urge to serve someone, in what way would you like to provide help?
~ Are you grateful to your friends for their presence?

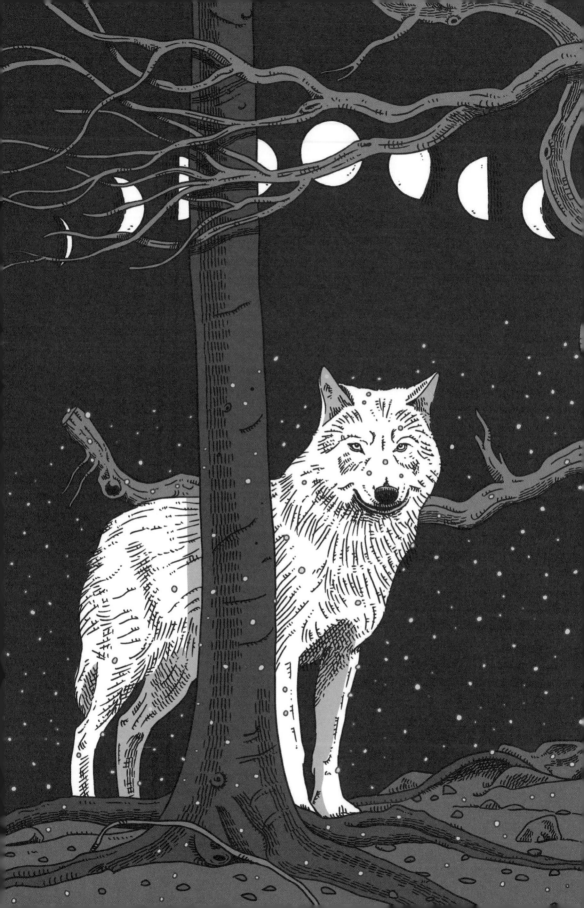

THE WOLF
The Wise One of the Mountain

Free, untamed, intelligent, the Wolf is the spiritual teacher who invites us to honor our innate wisdom. It is an animal sacred to the Moon, associated with the feminine creative force. It shows us the way to initiation, urging us to embrace our fears and overcome them with courage to understand our personal truth. For the Wolf explores, travels, and discovers who it is, experiencing the world. It knows where it comes from, and it also knows that to find itself it must leave its original pack and spend some time alone to acquire riches, only to return and make them available to all. True to its instincts and nature, it does not allow itself to be domesticated in exchange for comfort. With integrity, it chooses

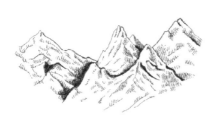

Embrace yourself in your wholeness, and wisdom will enter your Heart.

with whom to share its Life and creates a family it will care for until its death, but always staying true to itself. Sometimes its wild and domesticated sides are combined, to show us that beyond the division between light and shadow, between right and wrong, Life simply is, and cannot be caged. Its instinctive nature has made it a menacing and disturbing character in myths and fables. But the Wolf is the harbinger of a great awareness: our truth lies in the multiplicity of all our facets. Indeed, this animal teaches us how to embrace them and shows us how to hold them together, for it is in their union that the medicine of the Wolf is revealed to us.

AWARENESS QUESTIONS

~ Are you in touch with your wisdom?
~ What do you see in the people you choose as teachers that you don't yet see in yourself?
~ Do you recognize that everything and everyone can be teachers for you?
~ Do you nurture your wildest side?
~ Do you take care of yourself and of those you love?
~ Do you have faith in your instincts, or do you question them out of need for approval and validation?
~ Are fears an obstacle to your self-fulfillment?

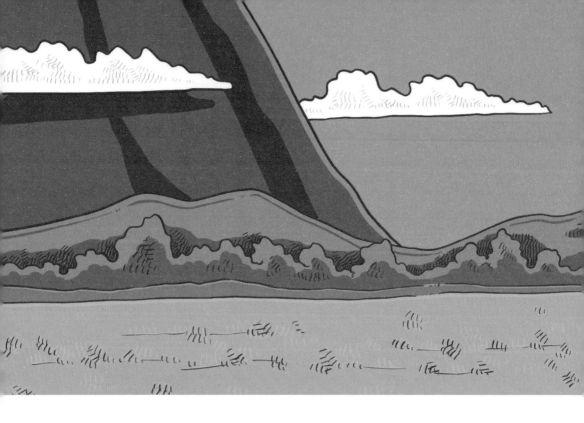

THE DONKEY
The Humble Servant

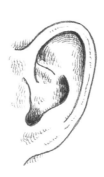

Z eus appointed the wise Titan Epimetheus to populate the Earth with animals, so he gave the Donkey to humans to help them with hard work, carrying heavy loads for them. The Donkey has always been a vital aid to humans, used both as a means of transportation and as a pack animal, especially in inhospitable and mountainous environments. Now that machines fulfill these tasks, they are

Humility is not submission or self-denial, but full acceptance of one's purpose.

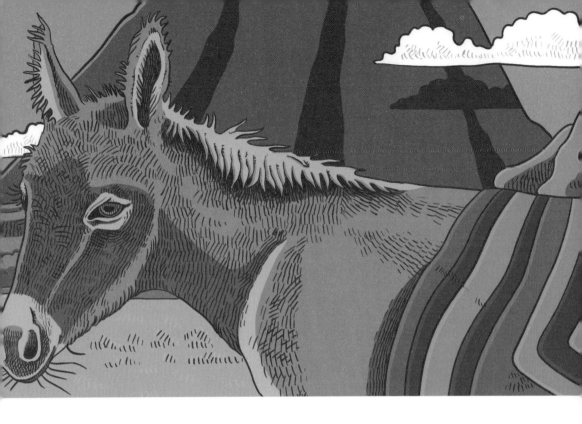

used for pet therapy and once again contribute to our well-being. The great service done to mankind reveals the humility that characterizes this gentle, sensitive, intelligent, determined, caring, wise, resilient, and reliable animal. With its large ears, it is a sensitive and attentive listener, sniffing out dangers at a great distance and keeping away from them. It tells us to ignore the opinion of others and to seek validation within ourselves, in the divine within ourselves. Often its humility has been read as stupidity: suffice it to say that the word "donkey" is used as an insult to define an ignorant person and that, until not so many years ago, students were humiliated in school by making them wear hats with fake Donkey ears. This simply reveals the limitations of human beings.

AWARENESS QUESTIONS

~ What does humility mean to you?
~ Do you feel humble?
~ How much importance do you attach to the opinion of others?

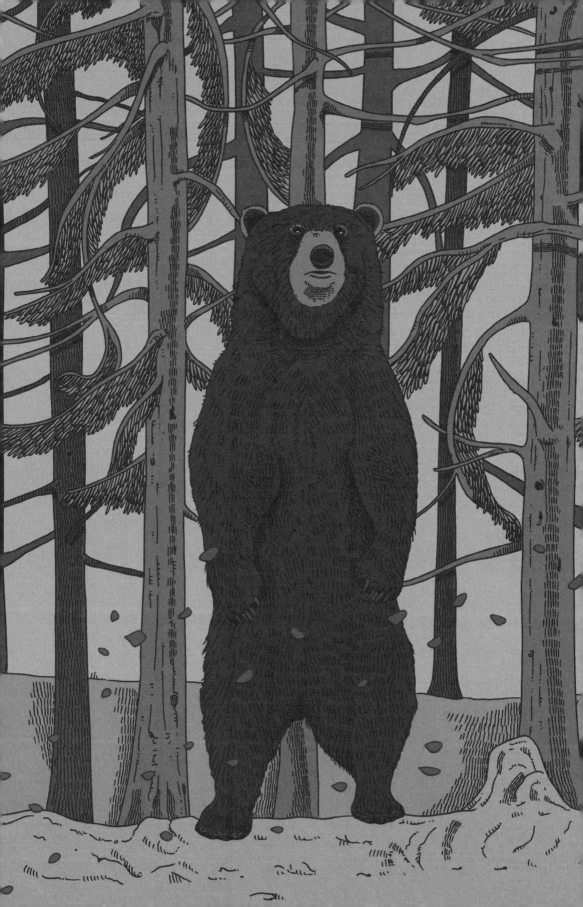

THE BEAR
The Power of Introspection

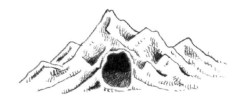

The Bear is a lunar animal strongly linked to the magic of silence, that place of inner peace that everyone can access and that allows us to stop and push away for a while all that is other and external. This large furry mammal that inhabits the pristine green lands, or the white expanses of ice, invites us to transmute solitude into conscious relationship with ourselves. It tells us that the answers to our questions will emerge in the silence of our inner cave, there where the power of the ancestors echoes and the pulse of Mother Earth is in tune and merges with our own. The Bear invites us to feel with the Heart, to descend into the depths of our very roots so that we can interiorize past experiences and learn a fundamental lesson: we know better than anyone else what is best for us. Spending quality time with ourselves, in fact, enhances our inner strength and our authority; it is vital to learn to know ourselves and others, and then consciously choose who we want next to us. Bears are wild, intelligent, strong, and protective animals, connected to the rhythms of nature, perfectly balanced between long introspective, lethargic periods, cocooned in the autumn/winter dimension of being, and other energetically open periods that instead they spend outside, active in the spring/summer dimension of doing.

> In inner silence you will find all answers. Learn to make solitude a time of deep connection with yourself.

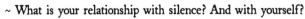

AWARENESS QUESTIONS

~ What is your relationship with silence? And with yourself?
~ Do you allow yourself to create spaces for introspection, listening, and welcoming?
~ Do you listen to your feeling, your innate wisdom?
~ In the silence of your Heart, what answer is waiting for you?

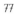

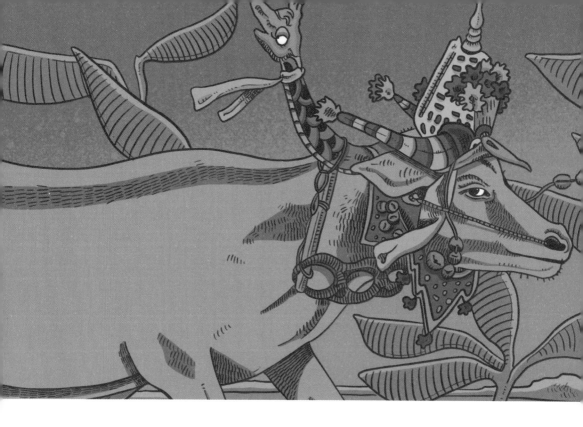

THE COW
The Cosmic Mother

A ssociated in all cultures with femininity, especially with respect to fertility, procreation, breastfeeding, and nurturing, the Cow or Sacred Cow is the one who nurtures with benevolence, love, and gentleness: all features of the Good Mother archetype. In Ancient Egyptian cosmogony, it is the first to emerge from the cosmic ocean of creation as Mehetueret, the Heavenly Cow, mother of all rebirths. Between its horns it carries the solar disk, initiating the temporal cycles of night and day, of death and resurrection; it gives birth to its son, Ra, each day so that light cyclically follows darkness on Earth. In art, the Cow's horns, symbolizing the female womb, will become the hallmark of all priestesses related to motherhood. In India, the killing of this animal was banned in 1527, and it is still

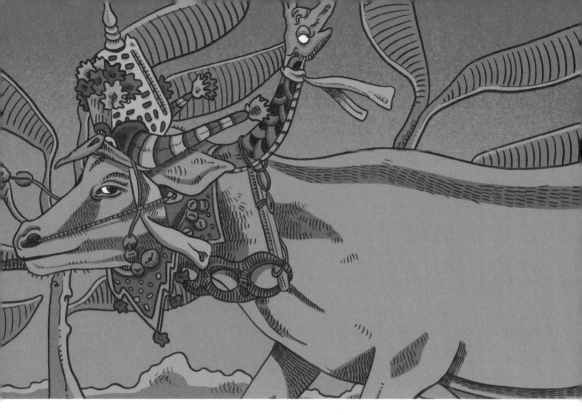

considered sacred and inviolable. With its large, soft eyes, the Cow invites us to let ourselves be nourished by experiences, savoring them calmly and slowly, fully in the moment, enjoying the possibilities offered to us. It encourages us to be maternal with all that is born of us, lovingly nurturing and protecting our creations. It also reminds us of the importance of taking care of the Earth and its natural resources, for it is through these that we can obtain our vital nourishment and ensure the survival of other species as well.

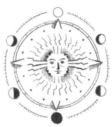

Everything that is born needs love, nurturing, and protection to grow.

AWARENESS QUESTIONS

~ Do you actively take care of natural resources?
~ Do you feel maternal with respect to your creations, your children? Do you take care of feeding, loving, and protecting them?
~ What is your relationship with the maternal sphere, with motherhood?

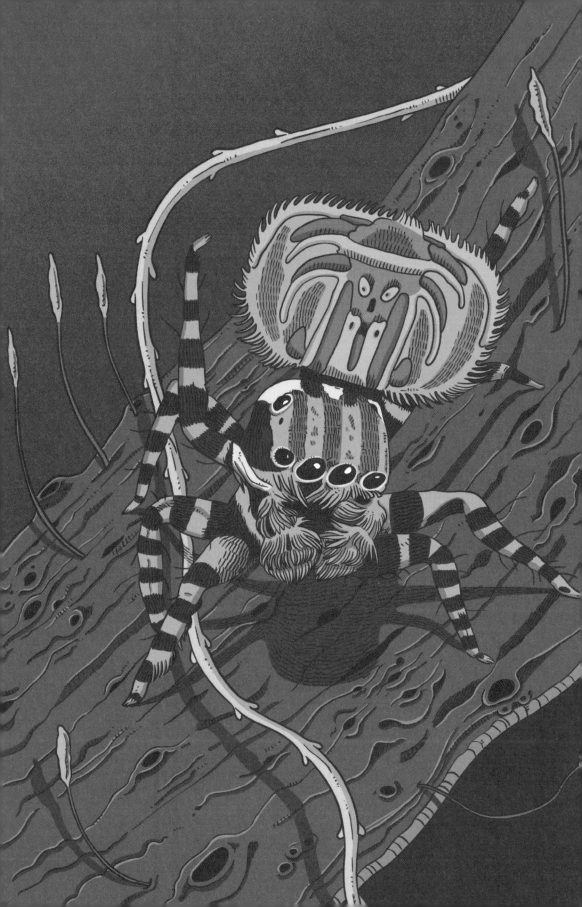

THE SPIDER
The Universal Weaver

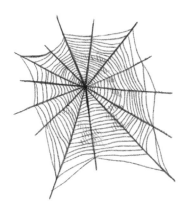

if we follow the cosmic force, of which we can be channels, our possibilities are endless. In actualizing the process of creation, the Spider reminds us that harmony arises from the balance of the parts, from the pure expression of one's talents, which weaving to the beat of the Heart generates beauty. As a weaver, the Spider is a symbol of patience, dedication, care, and endurance: all qualities needed to give life to something that did not exist before. However, in some it causes phobias, and it is usually associated with intrigue, crippling illusions, and cages that prevent progress.

W eaving divine webs of unspeakable beauty, the Spider symbolizes the female creative force that generates the forms of the world. There are several myths in which this arthropod creates the universe by weaving it. The Spider symbolizes the infinite possibilities of creation, our divine opportunity to design ways of Life, dwellings, professional and educational structures, as well as new languages to express ourselves and communicate. It reminds us that we can rework old models to shape new ones, more suited to our needs. It tells us that

I weave and unweave the canvas of my days, making my creation a work of art.

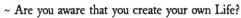

AWARENESS QUESTIONS

~ Are you aware that you create your own Life?
~ What do you want to create in the time you are given?
~ Do you feel free, or imprisoned, in fears and illusions that hold you back?
~ Do you celebrate your own creations? How do you relate to others' ones? Can you rejoice in them?

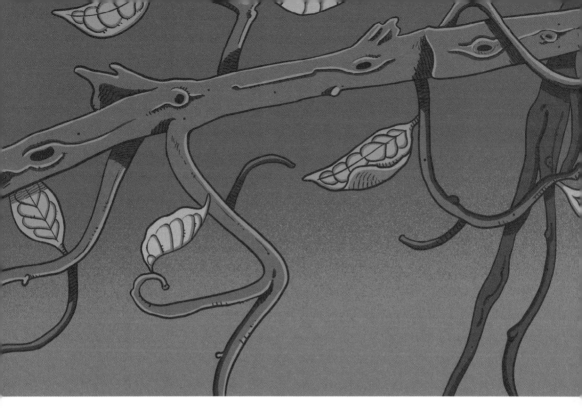

THE POSSUM
The Art of Surprise

I f there were an Oscar prize for animals, the role of best actor in a leading role would undoubtedly be awarded to the Possum. Its most important and unique characteristic is its ability to play dead when it is attacked and does not wish to fight, or feels there is no other choice. Then, this cunning creature shows all its acting skills by throwing itself to the ground, apparently stone-dead. During this performance, Possums are even able to lower their body temperature, simulate a death grimace on their faces, and even spray a liquid with a horrible smell of putrefaction from specific glands.

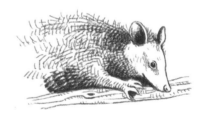

There is always a Plan B, an alternative solution, an ace up your sleeve.

82

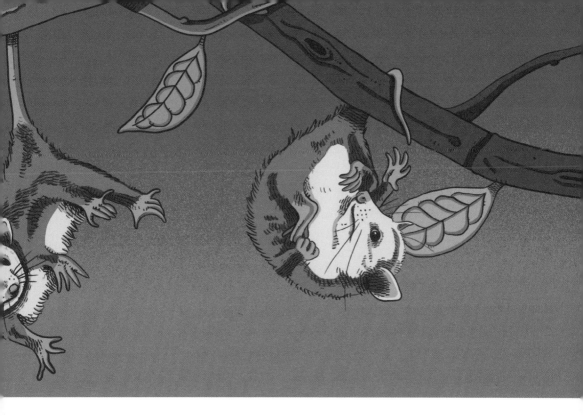

Their predators, believing them dead, loosen their grip, and the Possums, taking advantage of their distraction, flee. They are therefore very smart animals, which can also adapt to eating a wide variety of different foods and to living in very different environments. They always find an alternative solution when the situation turns out to be different from what they had expected. Their medicine is the art of surprise. Indeed, the Possum urges us not to give up surprising ourselves by drawing on unexpected resources, and to spare our energy by avoiding unnecessary fights, instead focusing on what really counts. It also teaches us to react cunningly when attacked.

AWARENESS QUESTIONS

~ What are the strategies you put in place when attacked?
~ Can you defend yourself when it is necessary to do so? Do you know instead when to avoid a battle?
~ Do you like to surprise people?
~ Do you let yourself be surprised?

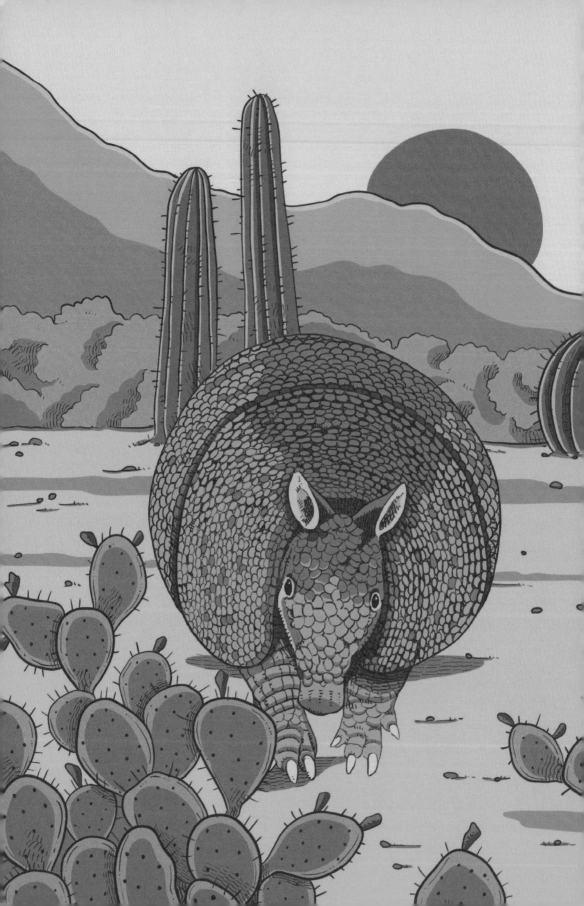

THE ARMADILLO
Setting Personal Boundaries

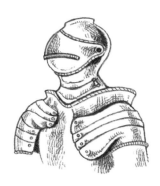

Armored with scales that look like those of a dragon, Armadillos roll themselves into a ball when attacked by a predator, creating an impregnable fortress. This armor-clad mammal that moves slowly, cautiously, and alertly, tells us about the importance of protecting our boundaries. It is a symbol of security and self-preservation, and like the Possum it reminds us of the importance of defense strategies. It is a peaceful animal that, instead of fighting, prefers to dig for food. If it does not find any, however, it is able to live several days fasting because of its resilience. The Armadillo embodies our primary need for security, and invites us not to feel invaded, abused, or outraged. Personal boundaries are sacred and mark our intimate, private space: everyone has the right to choose who can and cannot enter. Sometimes they are physical spaces, but they are often linked to our emotions, our mind, and our Soul, so learning to protect them is of paramount importance to living a free and peaceful Life. If we know when and from whom to protect ourselves, we will avoid various forms of abuse, as well as unjustified fear and distrust. The Armadillo encourages us to explore our boundaries, to set them so that we can protect them, and at the same time urges us to respect the boundaries of others and to always ask permission when we feel we are about to cross them.

know when to say "Yes" and when to say "No." I know that my boundaries are important, and therefore I protect them.

AWARENESS QUESTIONS

~ What do your boundaries look like? What do they protect?
~ Can you respect the boundaries of others?
~ Can you say "Yes" when you feel it is "Yes," and "No" when you feel it is "No"?
~ Do you wear armor even when you don't need to?

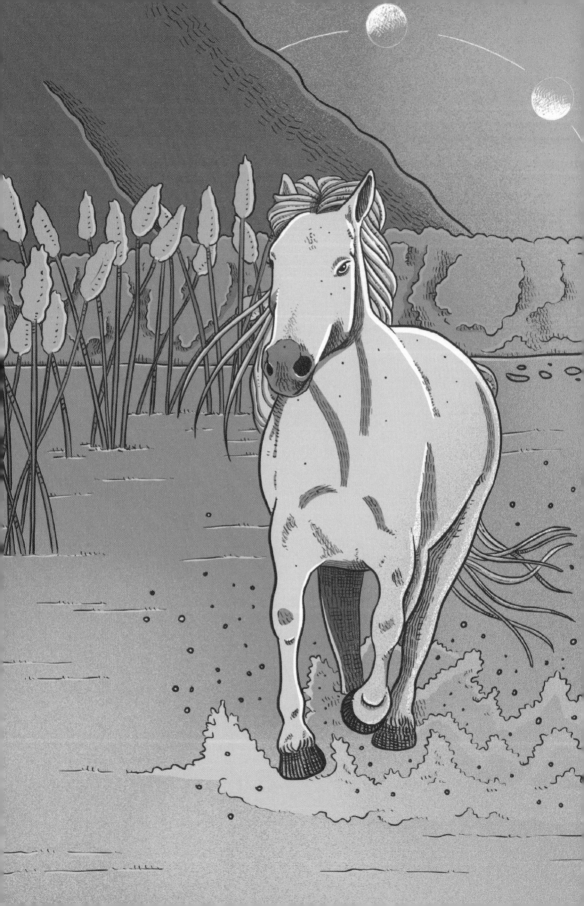

THE HORSE
The Free Spirit

Strong, elegant, and swift as the wind, the Horse is a symbol of freedom, power, and the nobility of Spirit. Deeply rooted in our earthly dimension, physical and spiritual at once, it has always accompanied knights, warriors and rulers, armies, and priests and deities in this and other worlds. A psychopomp (in Ancient Greek, the word means "an entity who escorts the souls from Earth to the afterlife"), this animal is linked to both lunar and solar aspects of the Spirit, and has always been associated with wealth, valor, merit, and prestige. For man it has been a faithful companion, an unquestionable helper, and a clear metaphor for the spiritual need to be free, wild. A Horse running alone or in a herd across a vast prairie is a clear symbol of Freedom. By allowing itself to be ridden, it has also given

The freedom to be yourself is a necessary condition for well-being, for embracing happiness.

humans the ability to travel at speeds otherwise impossible to achieve, thus almost certainly inspiring all modern means of transportation. Horses are intelligent, extremely sensitive, sociable, long-lived, and hard-working animals. Loyal to their companions, they can establish a deep emotional connection with their caregivers. The Horse invites us to let our hair down—the wind ruffling it—and run barefoot. It urges us to free ourselves from everything that hinders us and hides our true nature; to raise our arms to the sky and affirm our existence in the world.

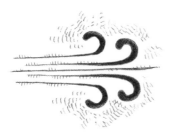

AWARENESS QUESTIONS

~ Do you feel like a Free Spirit?
~ How important is freedom to you?
~ Is being yourself too difficult or are you beginning to embrace your inner self?

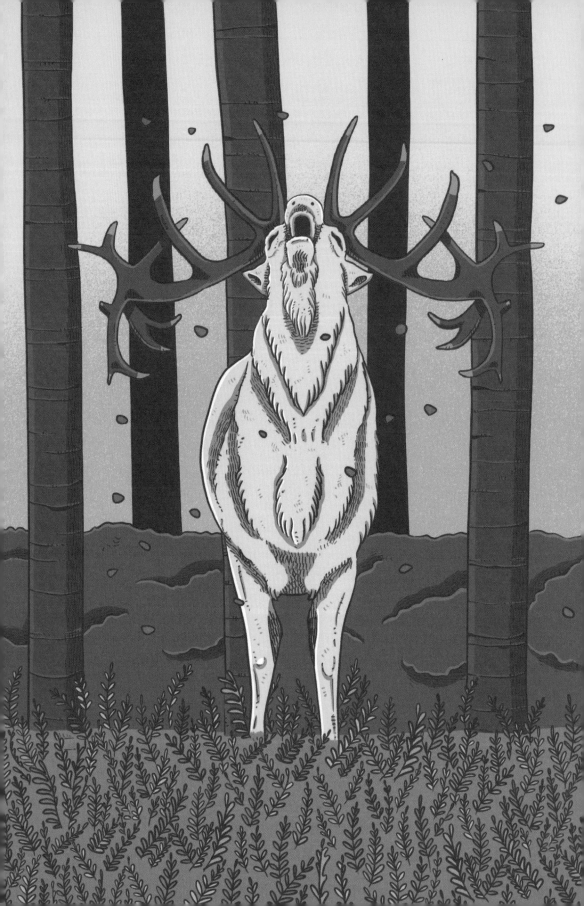

THE DEER
The Guardian of the Forest

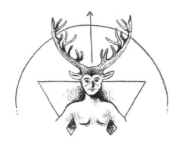

A symbol of royalty, dignity, poise, strength, and courage, the mere presence of the Deer expresses its proud belonging to nature, and with its head held high it takes on the role of its guardian. Although it is prey, it has the attitude of a predator, and it is difficult to catch because it is fast and a true expert in self-defense. Perhaps this is why in the Celtic Beltane fertility rites, when the sacred hunt was launched, the animal to be caught was the Deer, so that the hunter could prove his stubbornness and valor. It is a very peaceful creature, fighting only in late spring with other males to mate with the females. This is helped by its large horns, which like trees have their own cycle: they fall off in winter after the mating season and grow back in spring. They have been held sacred since prehistoric times, and in Celtic mythology Cernunnos, the lord of the forest representing the divine in nature, wears them. Shamans have always used them in their rituals, seeing in this animal a conduit to the divine and dream world. The Deer teaches us to become aware of our deep connection with Nature, of the coexistence of the following different spheres, inherent in us: divine, spiritual, wild, material, and magical. It invites us to be the guardians of our own Life, to protect it, to honor it with a peaceful and regal Spirit. It also urges us to strive only for that which allows Life to be preserved and ensures its continuity.

You must fiercely guard your treasures with an open Heart and a calm mind.

AWARENESS QUESTIONS

~ Do you have the pride of those who feel they belong to nature? Do you express it by walking tall?

~ What aspects of your Life and existence in general do you feel you are a guardian of?

~ What does nature represent to you? What about your relationship with it?

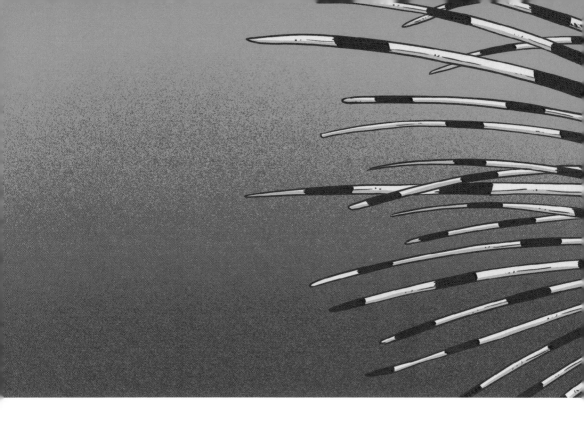

THE PORCUPINE
The Gentle Touch

The Porcupine is like a thorny thistle plant, which does not sting when touched gently. It teaches us the importance of our personal touch, and of the way we approach and relate to others. It makes us reflect on the fact that our kind or aggressive attitude generates different responses in others, resulting in openness or closure, in defense or attack. The porcupine is indeed a spiny animal, able to protect itself with its own body like the turtle and the armadillo, but it does so only when threatened. The spines are its own hair, which, when

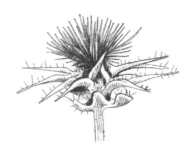

If you are kind, gentle, and sweet, your Heart will show you the way.

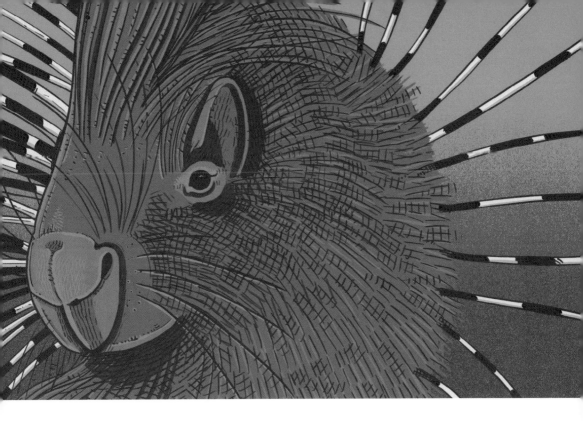

bristling, make its body look bigger and more dangerous: an excellent strategy against predators. Despite its outward appearance, its nature is neither unwelcoming nor pricky at all; it has instead a peaceful, playful, and friendly attitude and comes out mainly at night, illuminated by moonlight. The Porcupine teaches us to have faith in our own qualities, in our ability to take care of ourselves and at the same time in fate, knowing that Life always presents us with challenges that we have the resources to face. It invites us not to be intimidated by those people who seem repulsive and sullen, because even they hide an inner child who wants to play and be heard. They only show their spines because they are hurt and need to protect themselves. Instead of threatening them, we can approach wounded people with a very gentle touch and with sweet, sincere, and reassuring words.

AWARENESS QUESTIONS

~ When someone is prickly with you, do you attack them feeling hurt in turn, or do you use gentleness to reach out to them?

~ Are you aware that when you activate your spiritual 'spines,' you do so because you feel hurt and need protection?

~ Have you learned to gently touch the wounds of others?

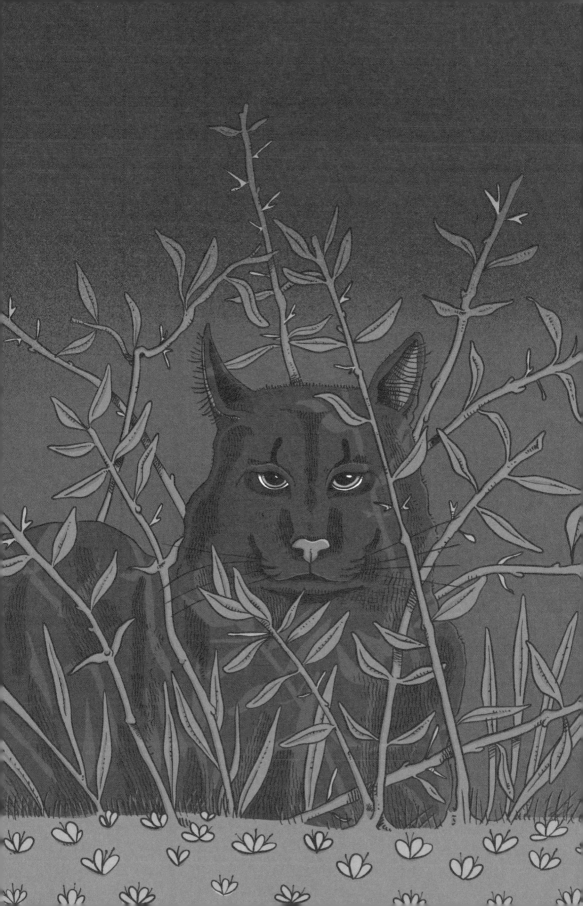

THE PUMA
The Leader

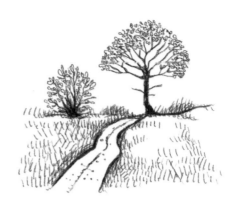

Elegant, agile, and quick, the Puma is a large black feline that embodies the strength of the mountain and the brightness of the polestar. The Puma is clearly born to be a leader. Life itself endowed it with the qualities needed to take on this role, in which personal power is intertwined with leadership. And although it is not easy to keep these two forces in balance, when we work hard on ourselves and spontaneously accept this challenge it comes naturally, because it is simply part of our path. Leaders must know how to take care of themselves and others, respecting everyone's process so as not to become the distorted projection of a parent, to whom people delegate their own duties and personal power. Knowing how to respect everyone's process does not mean saving people,

Leading others means taking on great responsibilities: this is the core value of a leader.

but rather helping them find what they need to accomplish the task on their own. They will come out stronger, centered, and in their full power. Leaders who have chosen ego over Soul, who still have too many wounds to heal, will create subordinates instead of collaborators; they will act unfairly for their own benefit; and instead of bringing light, they will cast a shadow on the Lives of others.

AWARENESS QUESTIONS

~ Do you feel that being a leader is part of your path?
~ Do you recognize yourself as a leader even in small groups, such as family?
~ If you are, can you respect the will of others, or do you impose yourself as a tyrant?
~ Are you avoiding the responsibilities that come with a leadership role?

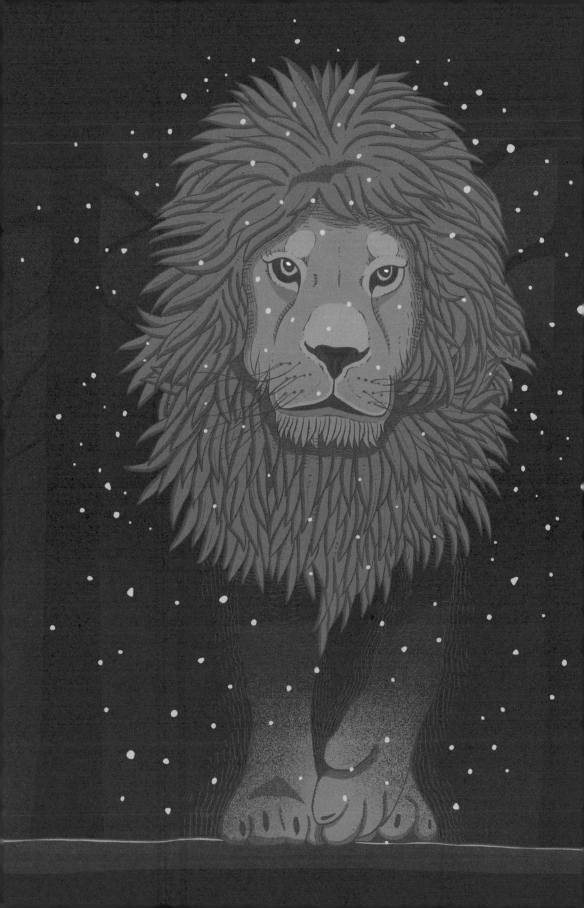

THE LION
The Ruler

The proverbial "king of animals," with its thick mane and confident expression, the Lion has become a symbol of kingdoms, lineages, and states. It is found, in fact, in many coats of arms and flags as a symbol of dominance, wealth, power, and authority. In the zodiac, this sign is linked to the Sun and expresses all solar power, embodying masculine creative force. It is the archetype of the ruler, of one who takes the lead of an entire people or nation and must have greater alignment with cosmic consciousness than others. As an inner archetype, it represents the wise, centered, rooted, and connected force within us, who can take risks and responsibilities for the greater good.

> I learned to be brave by facing challenges, and fear turned into inner strength rather than physical force.

Leo invites us not to be afraid to show ourselves for who we really are, which means to shine in our most intense and purest light. It tells us to recognize our spiritual kingship, the divine in ourselves, and to act accordingly, moving through the world as kings and queens who, in a continuous process of shadow integration, are constantly connected to the Heart and, from this state of mindfulness, manifest their power. It spurs us to serve our kingdom with our talents and gifts, ceasing to delegate our personal power to others, or lowering the intensity of our light. Leo urges us not to oppose our strength and beauty, but to put them at the service of all.

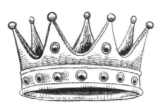

AWARENESS QUESTIONS

~ Do you feel like the ruler of your own Life?
~ Are you a Lionheart, meaning a strong, decisive, and courageous person?
~ In being a ruler, is the solar force of your Soul guiding you?

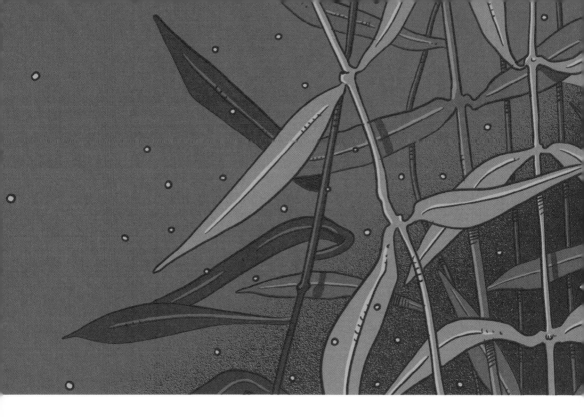

THE TIGER
The Independence
of the Warrior

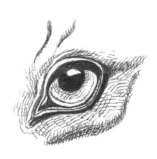

T he Tiger is a stubborn, patient, and constant predator. It waits until nightfall to hunt its prey and does not give up if it does not hit its target on the first try; in fact, it is even able to wait hours before achieving its goal. Among felines, it is the loner of the species, hunting and protecting its territory by itself. Characterized by strong individualism, independence is its totemic medicine. In Indian myths, it is an attribute of Durga, Kali, Bhairava, Kartikeya, and Narashima, warrior and protective deities, through whom it symbolizes inner strength. The Tiger invites us to become centered, free, independent adults who can take care of themselves and their needs. Independent adults know themselves, know what their needs are, and can act to meet them; they do not delegate their well-being and tasks to others, but take responsibility for them. Likewise, they do not take the needs of others upon themselves and do not create dependent relationships

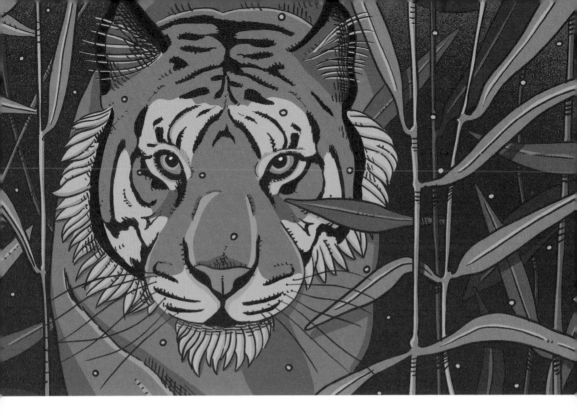

with other individuals. If developed too early, independence can be the consequence of emotional and psychic wounds in the child, who interiorizes the message that he or she must do it alone, that he or she cannot ask for help and trust others. In this case, it can become a trap leading to loneliness; by integrating the ability to ask, however, it becomes an exceptional strong point.

I relate, but I don't depend on anyone, and no one depends on me, because I am a self-fulfilled and complete being.

AWARENESS QUESTIONS

~ Do you feel like an independent adult?
~ How much does it matter to you to be one?
~ Are you able to ask in time of need, or do you have to make it on your own at all costs?
~ Are you enhancing your inner strength?

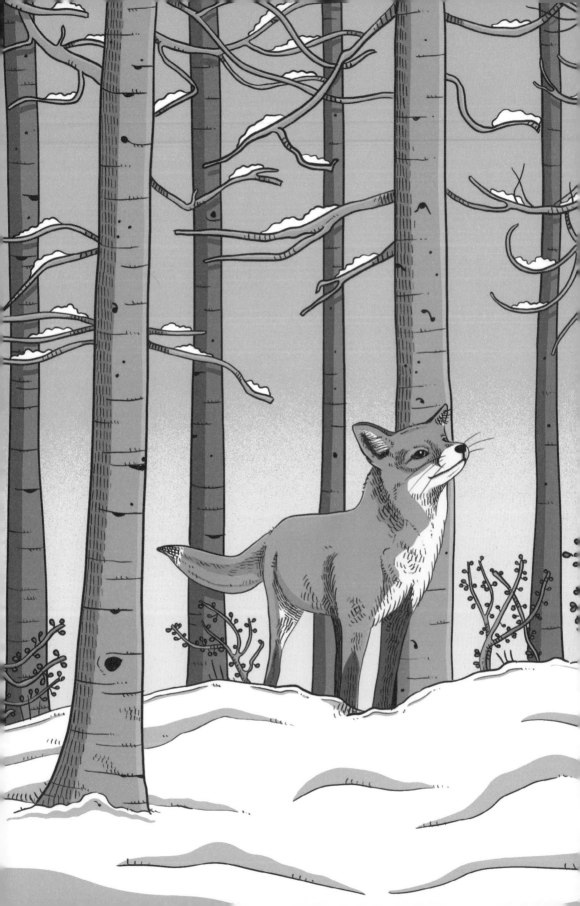

THE FOX
The Wiliness

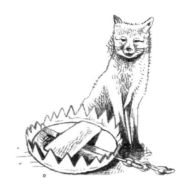

With its thick fur displaying typical autumn colors, in popular culture the Fox is associated with shrewdness and craftiness, even in a derogatory sense, referring to those who use malice and manipulation. In Norse mythology, for example, it is related to the god Loki, a symbol of deception; while in Chinese mythology it is linked to Daji, a concubine of King Zhou considered evil and a liar. Suspending judgment, we find that the Fox's medicine is wiliness, a skill it uses to go unnoticed and undisturbed as it progresses toward its goals. It invites us to do the same, to practice our creativity, to smoothly adapt to the sudden twists and turns of Life, with the irreverence of those who revel in difficulties. It offers us a very valuable medicine that transmutes complaint into creative force. The Fox is smart, intuitive, strategic, resilient, independent, and quick in thinking and acting; it welcomes the unexpected and plays with it, makes itself invisible to those who get in its way, and mocks adversity. It knows that unpredictability is part of Life and dances with it, making it fun and playful. It invites us to be like the wind, to learn with grace and a light heart to face every issue, going beyond appearances and relying on intuition.

I make myself invisible to those who hinder my growth, because I have no time to waste but goals to achieve.

AWARENESS QUESTIONS

~ Can you take Life as a game?
~ When you are faced with a difficulty, do you tend to stress, or enjoy yourself?
~ Are you able to come up with creative solutions, or do patterns guide you?
~ Can you be astute, or do you look at this quality with prejudice and reject it?
~ Do you adapt easily to sudden changes?

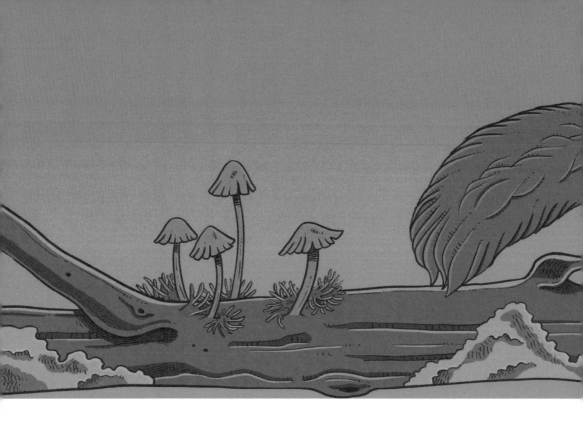

THE SQUIRREL
The Careful Collector

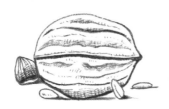

T he Squirrel is tiny, but it embodies a great medicine, namely the art of knowing how to collect and then store resources. It is a graceful and active rodent, often seen munching on its beloved nuts, climbing trees, or jumping very fast from branch to branch. Its thick tail allows it to glide,

I allow myself to receive
with immense gratitude
from Mother Earth
what I need, and when
I take more than
what I need,
I share it with love.

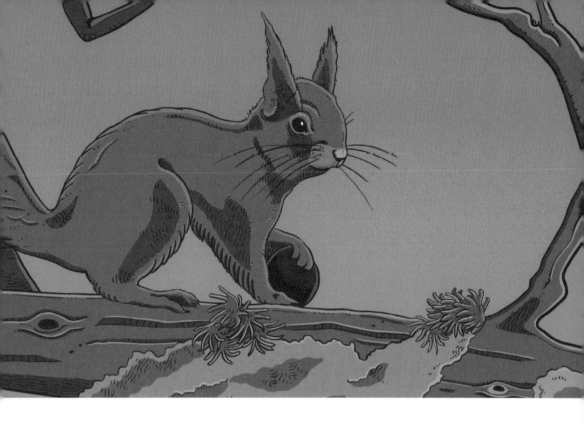

controlling its speed and direction. Its wingless flight inspires awe and wonder in anyone lucky enough to spot it. It's a wise little fellow: it knows that winter will come and so summer's abundance is not to be wasted. It does not hoard out of fear of scarcity and lack, but out of a deep respect for Mother Earth. Knowing her natural cycles, it actively takes part in them. It teaches us how to relate to abundance and shows us how to prepare for the future through a forward-looking approach to the cyclical nature of time. It invites us to collect and store energy, resources, knowledge, and money for when we need them and to consciously choose what we want to keep with us. The Squirrel accumulates its supplies in safe, protected places, sheltered from those who might take advantage of them; and this is an invitation to do the same, so that our labor is not in vain.

AWARENESS QUESTIONS

~ What do you need to store for the future you want to build?
~ Are you able to gather what you need?
~ When what you have gathered is too much, do you know how to let it go?
~ The 7 Chakra Crystals Proofread pages Are you able to share, or do you crave possession, show attachment to material goods, and want to keep everything for yourself?

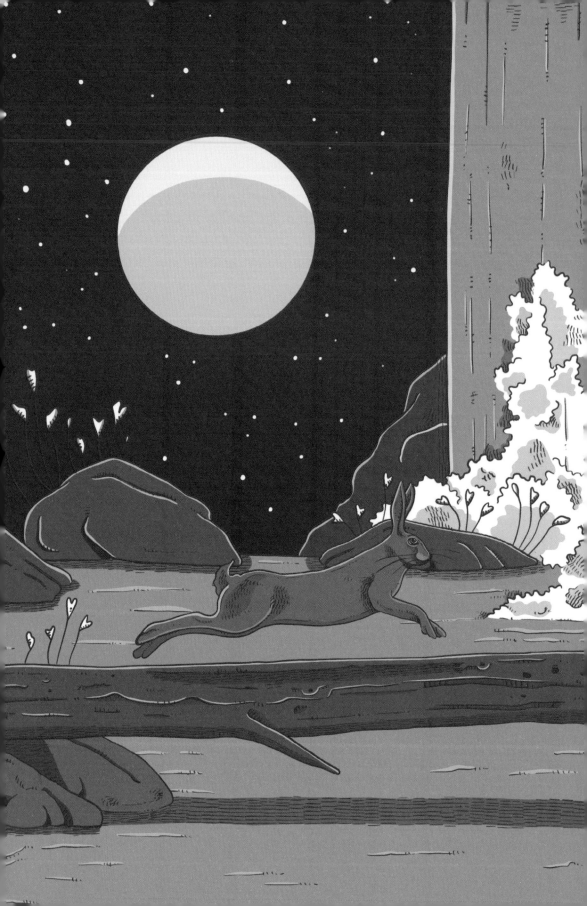

THE HARE
Fertility

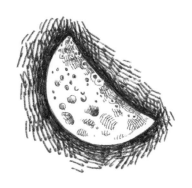

An attribute of Eostre, the solar goddess overseeing the spring equinox, the Hare symbolizes the fertility and fecundity of the Earth and is linked to the crescent phase of the Moon and thus to the East, the pre-ovulatory phase, as well as to the archetype of the maiden in the female medicine wheel. It is an attribute of new beginnings, of Life awakening to complete the journey from seed to bud, leaf, and flower, which in the coming season will become fruit. The Hare is a quick, alert, shy, and resolute animal. Equipped with large ears and strong paws, it feeds only on grasses and moves stealthily under the moonlight. In a Taoist legend, the Hare that lives on the Moon, in the shade of a fig tree, crushes the herbs of immortality in a mortar. It is in fact a symbol of longevity, a quality often associated with fertility. It mates at different times of the year, and its litters are very numerous. When something startles the Hare, it stops running, hiding from predators which mainly detect movement, and watches attentively for the best time to escape. It invites us to let the renewing, fertile, and fruitful energy of spring flow through us, to open ourselves to the forces of creation by becoming its channels and sources of new Life ourselves.

I give life to everything the Earth wants me to generate. I make myself a nest for all the upcoming possibilities.

AWARENESS QUESTIONS

~ Do you feel as fertile as spring at this point in your Life? What about in others?
~ How much does the energy of new beginnings scare you?
~ Have you learned to embrace it?

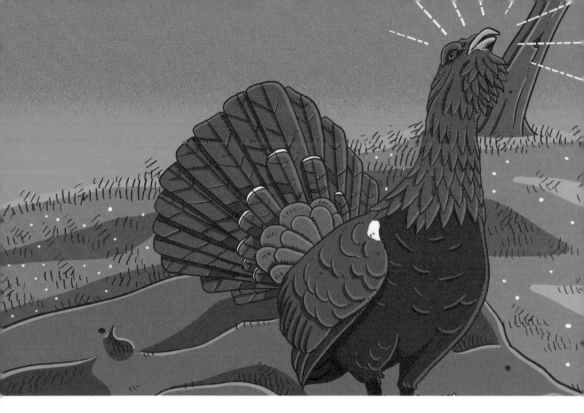

THE ROOSTER
The Daily Reminder

A ssociated with virility, masculinity, and vigor, the Rooster is the one who watches over, rules, and protects the henhouse. Like a sultan at the head of his harem. if it needs to defend its spaces and the chicks, it can become territorial and aggressive. It structures well-defined social hierarchies and gives its best performances during the mating season. Its courtship behavior somewhat made it the poster child of patriarchal masculinity. In an Ancient Greek myth, it oversaw the birth of Artemis and Apollo and was therefore

Some rituals mark time and help you remember what most counts. Use them to improve your memory.

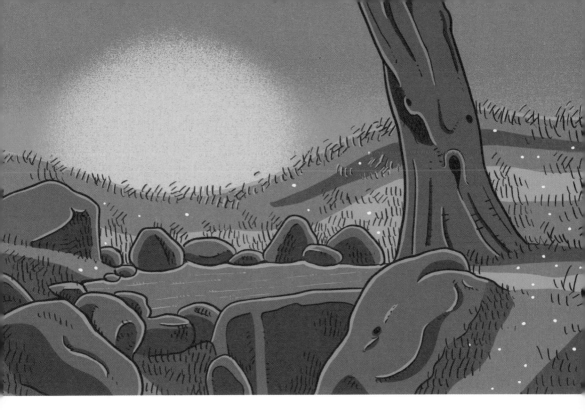

associated with both deities: the lunar and the solar one. It is no coincidence that, with its high-pitched crowing, the Rooster reminds everyone that night has given way to dawn, and that a new sun has risen. It invites us to be forward-looking, disciplined, to exercise control over our actions, and to pay attention to what is important to us. It encourages awakening and awareness of the present momen; and it tells us that it is no longer time to sleep, for a new time is upon us and awaits our contribution. It is a call to responsibility about the actions we choose to take on our journey.

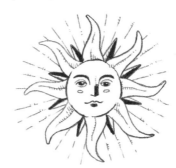

AWARENESS QUESTIONS

~ Are your daily rhythms marked by alternating light and dark?
~ Are you an early riser?
~ Do you mark your schedule on an agenda, or set the alarm clock as a reminder of your urgent tasks?
~ What is the best alarm clock for you?

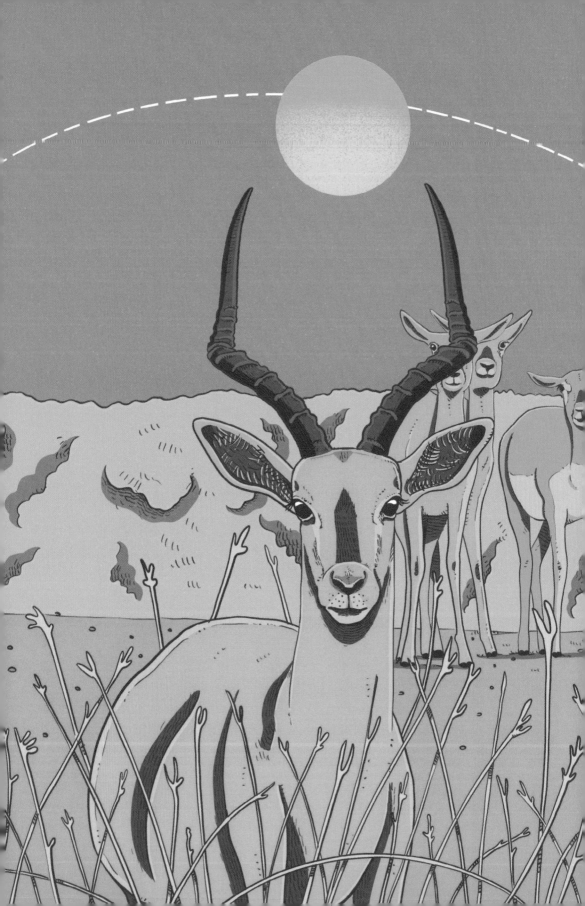

THE ANTELOPE
Acting Consciously

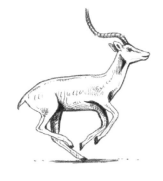

With its long, twisted horns, the Antelope grazes gracefully in large herds on the vast plains of Africa, Asia, and America. When it smells danger from large predators nearby, it wastes no time and quickly runs as far as it can. Its defense mechanism is precisely speed; and being prey, it uses it to escape. Antelopes are intelligent, knowledgeable, and energetic, and they can teach us how to use our resources and skills to survive and thrive, even in stressful situations. They invite us to be quick and agile in dealing with difficulties and obstacles, to focus on finding the solution to our problem as quickly as possible and implement it by making it a new opportunity.

> When I know what
> to do and go for it,
> all fears vanish
> in the light of awareness.

The Antelope tells us about action, movement, and consciousness, about deep listening and neutral observation of self and surroundings, of fear to be turned into strength, determination, and courage. This animal does not procrastinate, delay, or delegate. The moment it has clearly chosen what it wants to do, it simply acts. It's never hesitant or undecided between different options, because it knows the right action or movement to take. It internalizes, in perfect harmony, the voice of body, mind, and Spirit, which becomes one and guides it. In many cultures it has been associated with the ability to act responsibly, with physical strength and mental agility.

AWARENESS QUESTIONS

~ With the resources you have right now, what do you want to do in your Life, in the here and now?

~ When you know what to do, do you take responsibility to act?

~ If you had little time left to live, what would you absolutely do before you died?

~ What have you been putting off for so long?

~ Do you have a direction? What is the first step to take?

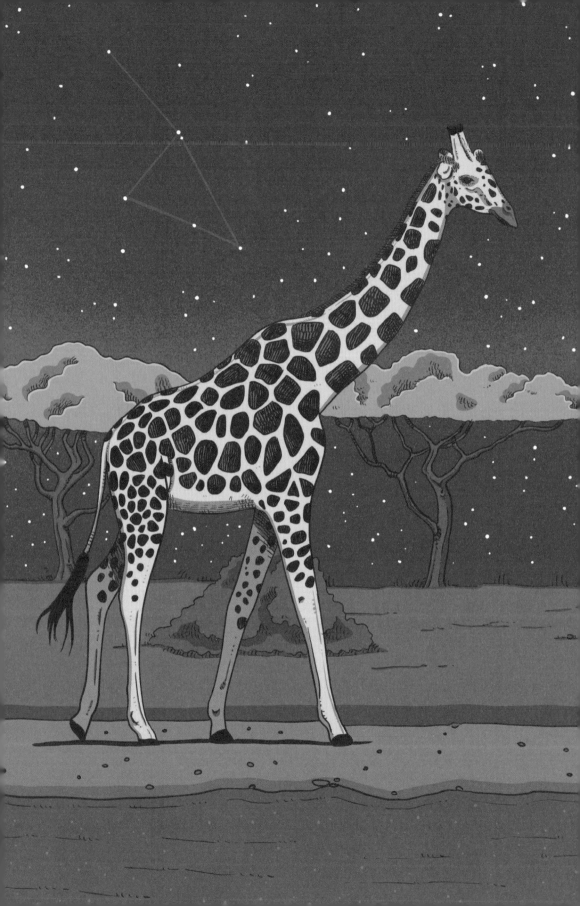

THE GIRAFFE
The Expansion of the Heart

Mild, peaceful, and running free in the savannas, the Giraffe is an animal with very long legs and neck, considered in Africa a messenger of the gods, a bridge between heaven and earth, a harbinger of peace and harmony. In the Somali language, its name means "smile." This animal is defined by marked sensitivity, patience, intuition, and resourcefulness. With its very long neck, the Giraffe symbolizes the ability to rise, to be above any scarcity and misery, to attain the sweetness of grace, bliss, and heavenly love.

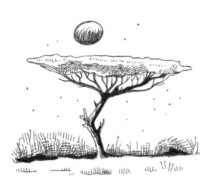

When Love within my Heart expands, I can reach great heights and embrace the Whole from a broader perspective.

This upward movement teaches us to look with the eyes of the Soul, enhancing noble qualities such as compassion, empathy, understanding, acceptance, nonjudgment, and kindness. Among land mammals, it is the one that possesses the largest Heart of all. This is why the Giraffe has become the symbol of Marshall Rosenberg's Nonviolent Communication, which is precisely called Giraffe Language, as it is expressed through the ability to empathize and give from the Heart. The Giraffe invites us to lift it up and walk the path of love with our heads held high, radiating all around us the wisdom of our Soul.

AWARENESS QUESTIONS

~ Is your Heart filled with love and thus expanding, or is it contracting, devoid of gratitude?

~ Do you feel free to walk tall, or do you carry burdens that prevent you from doing so?

~ What do you see, looking from the heights of the Soul?

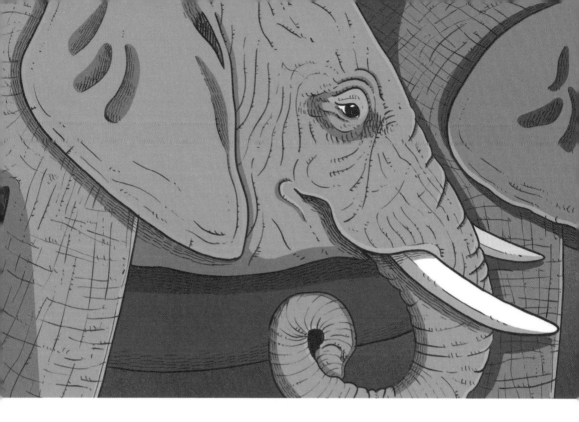

THE ELEPHANT
The Power of Vulnerability

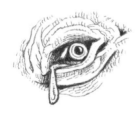

In India, they have a saying: "If you see everything gray, move the Elephant." Obviously, they chose this specific animal because of its huge size. Like humans, the Elephant is very long-lived, has an excellent memory, uses its strength very wisely, is protective of the vulnerable, and is curious, emotional, and empathetic. Self-aware, it recognizes itself in the mirror and shows sadness and grief at the death of another pack member. Its tears are often captured in photos, stirring up the same feelings of tenderness and compassion that it is in turn able to experience and feel. The Elephant invites us to validate all our emotions, even the uncomfortable ones, to normalize pain, sadness, and crying, because they are a sign that we have

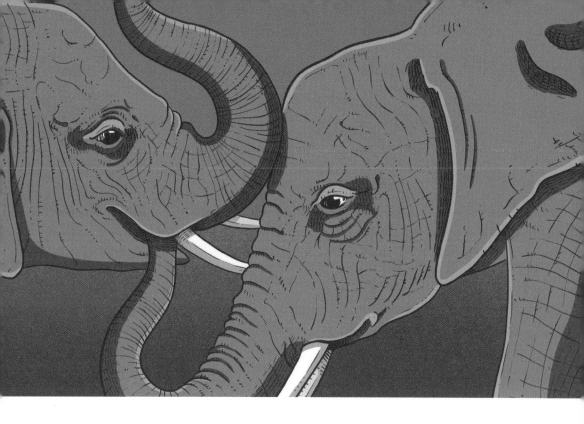

a beating Heart expressing a wide range of emotions: a Heart that is not withered by over-control and defense. It tells us that even a huge, strong being is capable of feeling emotions, which are entitled not only to small ones (children), but also to adults. This connection with our emotional side allows us to have good memory, to establish relationships, to experience the world through our own feelings, which sometimes match those of others: when this convergence is revealed, the magic of empathy happens.

Showing vulnerability and letting your emotions shine through is not weakness, but acceptance of yourself, of your life.

AWARENESS QUESTIONS

~ What is your relationship with your emotionality?
~ Do you allow yourself to be openly vulnerable?
~ Do you allow yourself to cry your heart out if you need to?

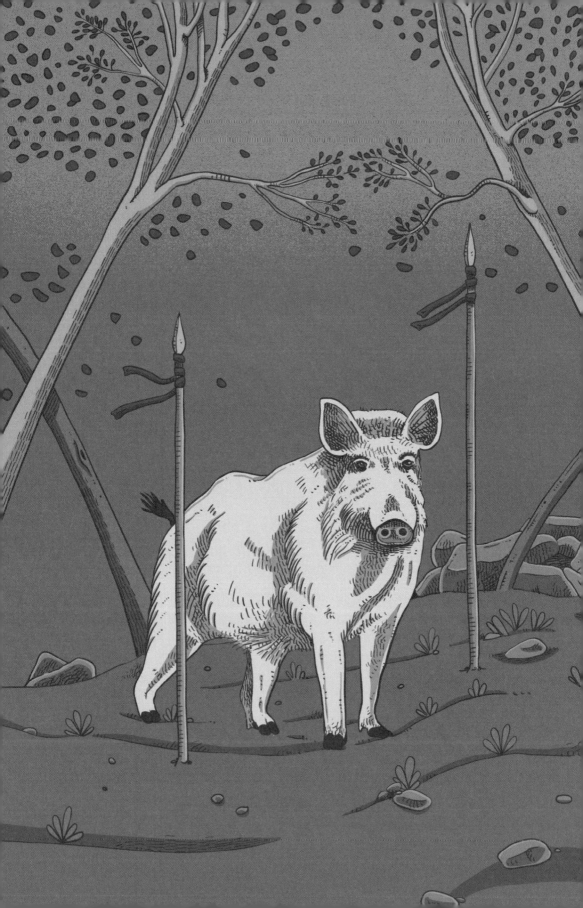

THE WILD BOAR
The Untamed Force

The famous "White Boar" sung by Franco Battiato, found in Celtic Druidic culture and Hindu mythology, symbolizes the spiritual awakening of every individual, the full consciousness of the physical and spiritual reality of the cosmos, which is free from illusions. Oddly enough, all this is embodied by an animal considered nowadays to be a destructive, troublesome pest, as its population has increased disproportionately given the shortage of its natural predators. For the Celts, the Boar was a valuable totemic ally to be taken with them into battle; and, to soak up its energy, its image was engraved on weapons and shields. In Greek myths, to give heroes worthy opponents, they were made to fight huge Wild Boars. Indeed, they represent endurance, revenge, the wild and brutal force that cannot be tamed. The Wild Boar teaches us how to summon the strength it embodies whenever we feel lost, disoriented, exhausted, or dull. It shows us that the way forward is our wild nature, connected to the woods, the forests, and the moist, dark earth. And when we receive its gift, it spurs us to protect it, lest we extinguish it again, for it is in wild contact with nature that our strength can be awakened and nurtured.

> When all seems lost, turn to your wild side and you will find the strength you need to refocus.

AWARENESS QUESTIONS

~ Can you be combative, proud, indomitable when the treasure to be protected is really important?

~ How much does your wildness scare you?

~ Are you actively working for the new advent of the "Era of the White Boar"?

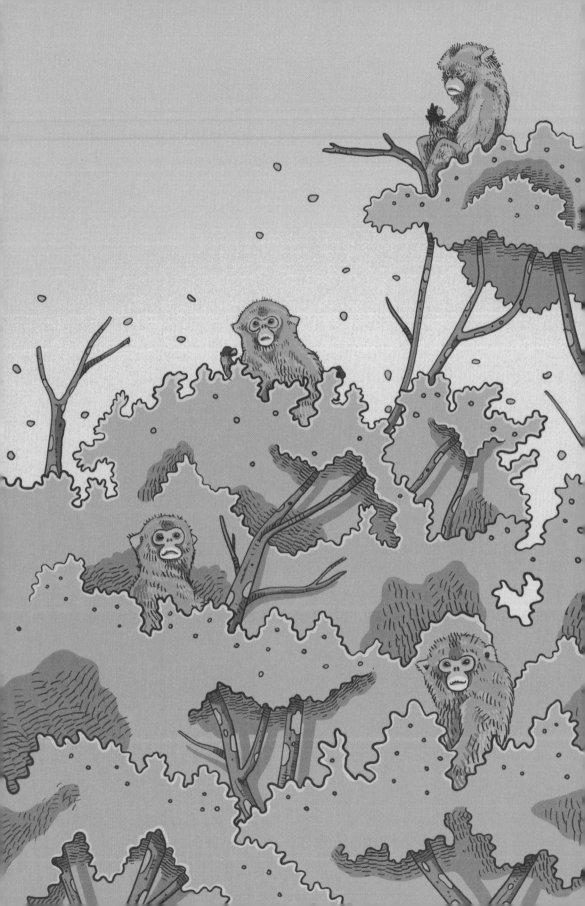

THE APE
The Curious Climber

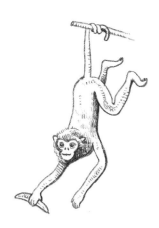

In the animal kingdom, the Ape is the most "human" creature in terms of appearance and behavior. Its intelligence and learning abilities are comparable to ours: in fact, it knows how to use tools, and it communicates and emotes like us. In Western culture, it is seen as the embodiment of primal impulses, capital vices, the lower self of man, governed by basic drives expressed without rules, order, and direction. Conversely, in the Buddhist tradition it is a symbol of intelligence, sensitivity, and ever-evolving consciousness, making it the wisest animal of all and therefore the one evolutionarily closest to man. The Ape is by nature playful, driven by a desire to explore, learn and know, has a childish sense of humor, enjoys playing pranks, loves to be in company, is creative, spontaneous, and often cheeky and irreverent. It invites us to increase our curiosity, reminding us that when we were children, Life was more fun, more enjoyable. Curiosity is essential to learn new things, to have experiences and adventures; without it, we could not climb tall trees, make new friends, or open ourselves to a new romance.

Curiosity will lead you out of the box, revealing unexpected amusements and allowing you to embrace the beauty you deserve.

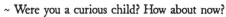

AWARENESS QUESTIONS

~ Were you a curious child? How about now?
~ Do you have self-control? How do you deal with your instincts?
~ Does curiosity represent a danger, or an opportunity, for you?

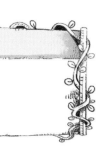

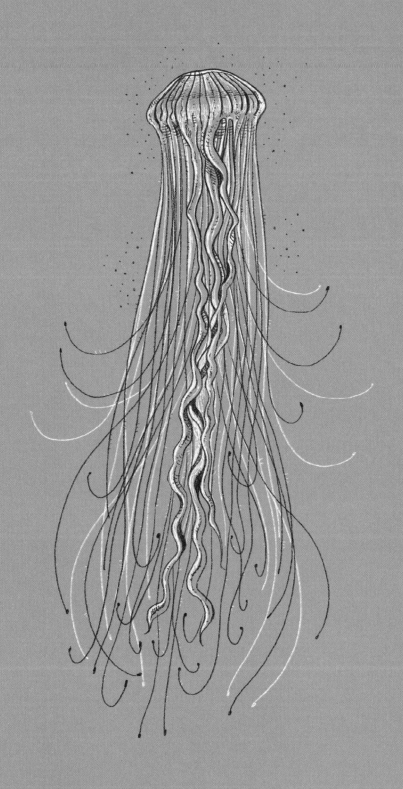

WATER ELEMENT ANIMALS

The Water Element Animals take us back to our Interiority, to our emotions, to everything inside us that is submerged, concealed, hidden, but not inaccessible. Water always finds a way to flow and reach its destination. These animals speak of movement, transitions, and trans-mutations; of strong currents followed by stagnation. They invite us to adapt, change, and explore what we consciously or unconsciously hold within ourselves. They remind us that we are much more aquatic than we think.

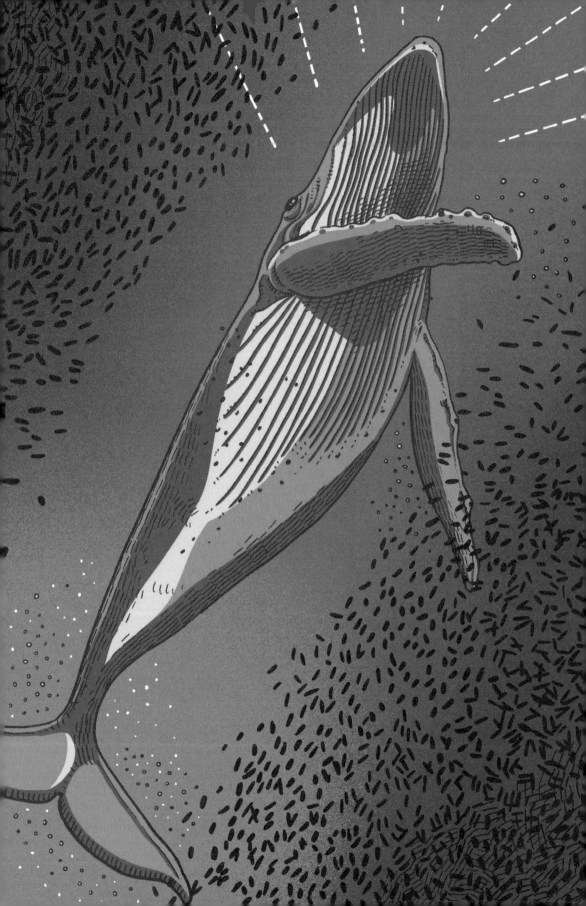

THE WHALE
The Keeper of the Akashic Records

T he Whale is the keeper of the ancestral memories of the Earth. It is a guide in the Akashic realms and, as such, allows us access to ancient knowledge. Its medicine is remembrance, and it invites us to disclose our inner space of silence, flowing past our emotions like clear water, to receive and channel knowledge. In Inuit culture it is seen as a powerful protector, a Spirit guide for fishermen, and is considered sacred, a spiritual conduit between the land and ocean worlds. With its large body, it swims

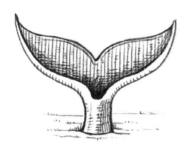

Find your sound,
your song,
and open yourself to the
knowledge of your Soul.

across all the planet's seas, from tropical to cosmic ones, and depending on the species it chooses its habitat. In many traditions and legends, including Buddhist ones, Whales are said to have stellar origins and to have appeared on Earth to help humans elevate themselves spiritually, to reconnect with their Soul. From time immemorial, the Whale offers the gift of its sidereal song, which is healing for our subtle bodies. It teaches us to use sound and frequencies as means of knowledge, to immerse ourselves in the spiritual energy of our Soul. This wise guardian embodies the immensity of our Higher self and tells us that we can reach it through song and silence. With its medicine, it invites us to find our voice and raise our song to heaven.

AWARENESS QUESTIONS

~ Have you found your song yet?
~ Do you express your voice fluently?
~ Do you allow yourself to delve into the depths of your existences, or are you afraid to know?

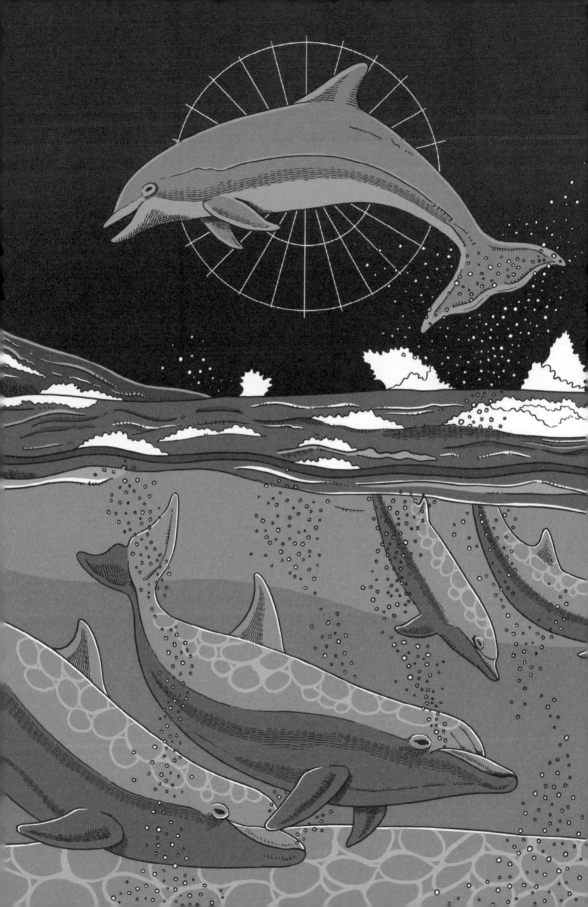

THE DOLPHIN
The Eternal Child

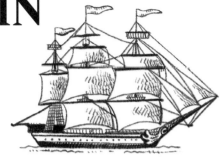

The Dolphin is a mammal that has always been considered a friend of man, an ally that can be trusted. It is, in fact, a leading character in all stories related to the sea, the great womb of planet Earth: as told by Homer, it was a dolphin—sacred animal and personification of the god Apollo—that led a ship of Cretan merchants to the place where the sanctuary of Delphi was later erected. Not surprisingly, the sanctuary's name is derived from *delphis*, "dolphin," which in ancient and modern Greek also means "womb."

> Repetition is an illusion. Live each moment for what it really is: always new.

It is linked to the inner child within us, or the vibrant and joyful energy of those who open themselves to adventure with playful enthusiasm. Forced to regularly surface to breathe, the Dolphin turns this need into an opportunity for fun and pleasure, to enjoy fresh air and explore the world from a different angle, opening itself up to encounters. It therefore invites us to develop a positive mental attitude so that we can look at difficulties as opportunities for discovery and growth, always in search of beauty. Because of its peculiar behavior, the Dolphin is associated with the breathing practices that are adopted along the spiritual path: thanks to its spontaneous and deep connection with breath, the Dolphin is, in fact, in a constant meditative state, which allows it to live in an eternal present.

AWARENESS QUESTIONS

~ Do you feel joy and gratitude for just being Alive?
~ Are you open to cooperation and altruism?
~ Are you connecting with your inner child? Do you allow yourself to have fun? Do you open yourself to pleasure?
~ Are you a spontaneous person?
~ Do you breathe consciously, descending into your depths and ascending to our surface?

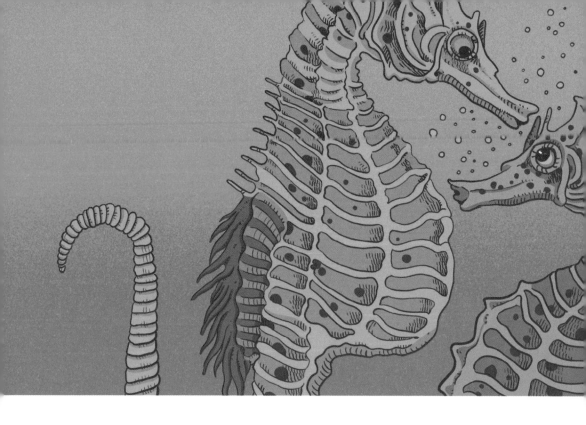

THE SEAHORSE
The Romantic Lover

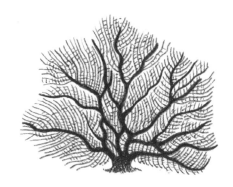

With its calm, patient, and relaxed disposition, this little sea dragon is a romantic, caring lover which chooses its mate and loves it for a lifetime. When one of them dies, the other does not seek a new mate, but devotes its Life to something else. According to a legend, the origin of the Seahorse, or Hippocampus, is quite bittersweet: two horses in love were chased by some hounds to a precipice over the sea; instead of giving themselves up to their pursuers, they chose to end their Lives by throwing

There are treasures so precious, so important, that when you find them, nothing else matters.

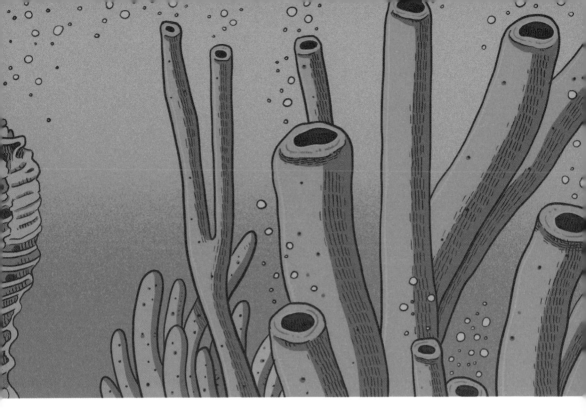

themselves into the water together; but as they plunged, something magical happened, and their bodies were turned into what we now all know as the Seahorse. Since then, as a tribute to that great love, all Seahorses live their romantic relationships with passion, deep union, and total fusion, creating a strong bond, a core that the couple honors and respects. Every morning, the two lovers dance, intertwining their tails to celebrate and reaffirm their Love. In the pair it is the male who gestates and gives birth—from a small marsupial pouch—to the countless eggs that the female has previously laid there.

The Seahorse teaches us to be caring, to cherish our most important humans, and to be loyal to our partner if we choose to be in a monogamous relationship. It tells us that the love of a couple must be nurtured, honored, celebrated with dances, and reaffirmed every day; that the partner must be chosen again and again to rekindle the couple's fire. Commitment, shared projects, and togetherness must be renewed.

AWARENESS QUESTIONS

~ What is your ideal type of relationship?
~ Are you willing to take care of the love you feel for others?
~ What characteristics should your partner have?
~ Do you like romance?

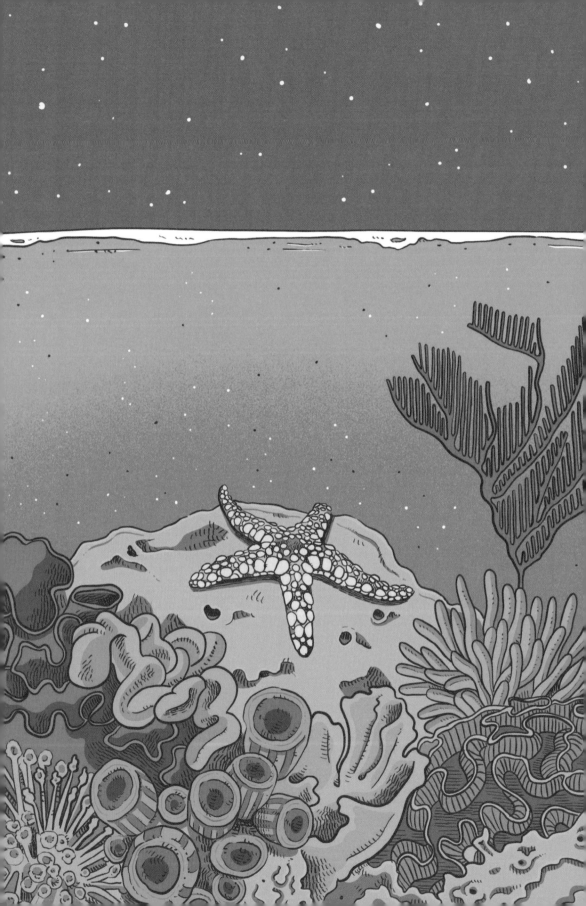

THE STARFISH
The Non-Attachment

With four, five, six, seven, or eight arms, on a full-Moon night, the stars fell into the sea to bring light and hope to the depths of the ocean. Attracted by the presence of Atlantis, they reminded its citizens that there were many worlds they had previously inhabited, including cosmic ones, and that the underwater city would be one of many others. They became a symbol of non-attachment, inviting people to flow with the currents of Life, and to practice letting go. Since then, they continue to convey this message in the crystal-clear waters of all the seas. Humans are captivated by these creatures, so much so that everyone, as soon as they see one, wants to take it, as if they had caught a star in the sky. But remember that if you take them out of the water, even for a

> Enjoy every drop
> of beauty
> in its uniqueness.
> More will come,
> in other places,
> but they will never be
> the same.

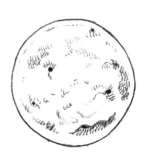

few seconds, their Life is endangered, just like the stars that shine above our heads; so look, don't touch. With its shape, the Starfish recalls the cosmic ocean of creation, reminds us that what is above is also below, that stars shine in the sky as well as under the sea. Like a mentor who accompanies us throughout our many existences, families, and experiences, the Starfish urges us to seek light in the darkness. It is an attribute of Venus, the sea-born goddess of beauty, who curiously enough is also a planet and has always been called the Morning Star.

AWARENESS QUESTIONS

~ In this existence, do you practice non-attachment?
~ Do you think you have only inhabited this planet, only worn this human form?
~ How attracted are you to the stars? What do they evoke?

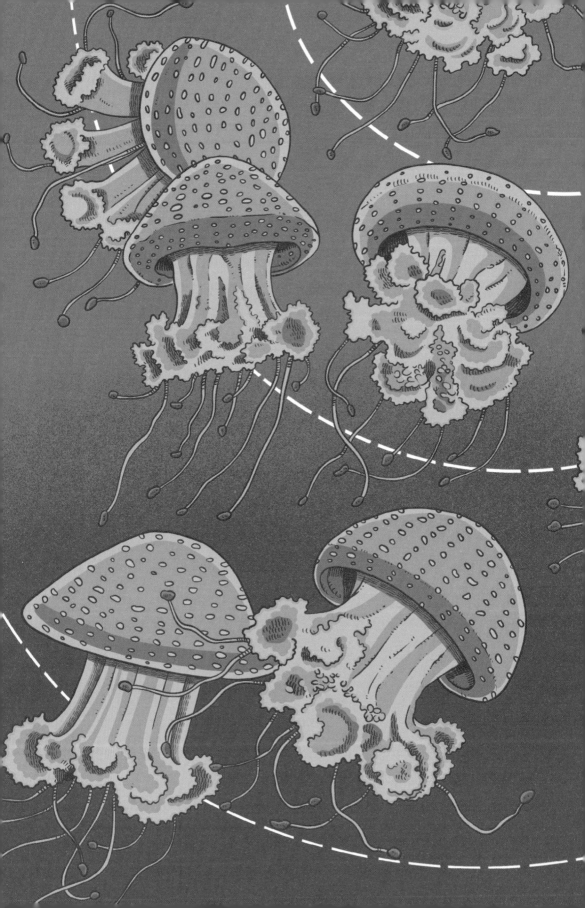

THE JELLYFISH
Flowing with a Light Heart

The Jellyfish is a very ancient animal that embodies a fundamental medicine: the ability to flow with the movements of Life, with the vital currents that move the whole universe. Learning to flow gives us the lightheartedness needed to live in harmony, to have a relaxed existence, free from contractions, worries, and obsessive thoughts. It allows us to gently let go of the past and lovingly open ourselves to the future. For this to be possible, what we need is trust, faith in Life. How could we trust someone or something unreliable? The Jellyfish will show us the way. It does not control its movements; it simply trusts and lets itself be carried by the current, flowing. It blends with the waves and becomes part of them. This is not because it cannot do otherwise; indeed, despite its excellent ability to swim and direct its body with its tentacles, it chooses to let go. Its tentacles are stinging, and if you come into contact with them, crossing the path of the Jellyfish, they can hurt. Its body, perfectly radially symmetrical, is transparent, not hiding what it contains; it invites us to make our mind as clear as its body, to create our personal inner space, letting go of worries and limiting beliefs that hinder our flow. The Jellyfish spurs us to embrace change with a confident, soft, and open Heart.

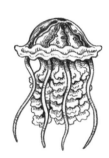

Clear your mind, meditate with a pure Heart, and trust the currents of Life. They will take you where you need to go.

AWARENESS QUESTIONS

~ In what ways do you approach change?
~ How much do you trust Life and yourself?
~ Are you able to rely on Life?

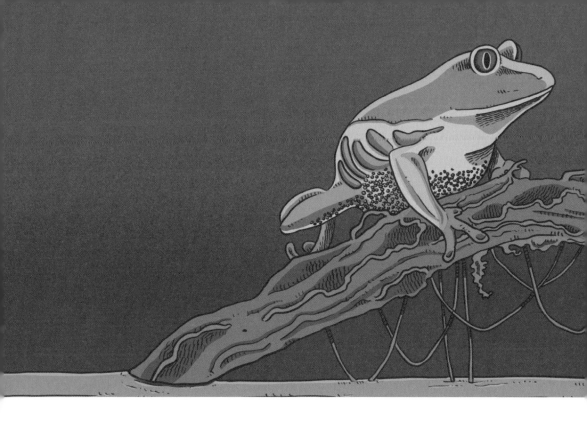

THE FROG
The Alchemist that Purifies through Water

A n amphibian that lives between the waters and the land, during its journey the Frog undergoes an evolutionary change that has, over the centuries, made it a symbol of adaptation, renewal, and protection. In ancient cults, primal female deities often had the likeness of frogs, an animal linked to fertility and childbirth, but also to creativity and regeneration. In Ancient Egyptian cosmogony, Heket, the frog-faced mother-goddess of creation, protected fertilization, birth, and rebirth after death. Frog-shaped statues dating

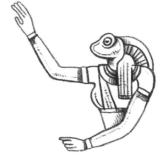

Purify yourself from what does not contribute to your well-being, and your life energy will be renewed.

to the Neolithic period have been found in Europe, Central Asia, and South America: their crouching position, with open legs and prominent vulva, harkens back to the natural position of women giving birth. The process of metamorphosis of this extraordinary animal can be likened to that of a human being: just like us, in fact, the Frog grows up in a watery womb until it is ready to leap out to experience

Life in new contexts, as fluid as the water where it was born. Its hypnotic-sounding croaking is an invocation to the heavenly waters to descend to Earth and enliven what has dried up, lest the mud solidify and become a trap. The Frog invites us to renew our energy and listen to our emotions, letting them flow: it teaches us to honor tears, the sacred water flowing from our bodies to purify us.

AWARENESS QUESTIONS

~ Do I accept the idea of renewing myself, getting rid of relationships, environments, and dynamics that do not give me peace and harmony?
~ Is there something that is drying up my energy?
~ Do I perform the actions needed to replenish my Spirit?
~ Do I allow myself to ask for help when I deal with forces out of my depth?

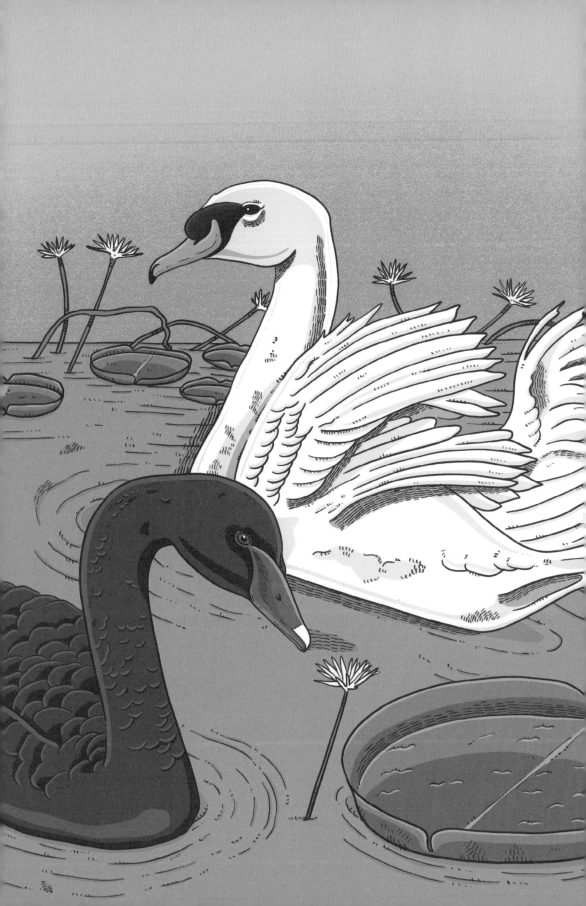

THE SWAN
Trust the Wait

Do you remember the story of the Ugly Duckling? In this fairy tale, the main character, which was seen as awkward and ungainly, gaunt, dark, abnormal, and misunderstood among the ducks, was actually a Swan undergoing its own transformation process. It was surrounded by unrelated souls that did not understand what was happening, because this metamorphosis was not part of their experience. Only by being patient, waiting for the process to be completed, will the ugly duckling become a wonderful Swan, graceful, elegant, and snow-white, and meet its true family. This story tells us about the alchemical process of transmutation and the need to trust in order to go through it and open oneself to grace.

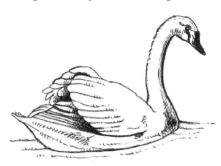

Be patient, trust the process you are going through: time will tell, and grace will come.

The swan is celebrated in many literary and theatrical works; and because of its physical characteristics, it has become a symbol of elegance, beauty, purity, and poetry. It swims in clean waters, and its whiteness makes it pleasing to the eye. It invites us to lovingly rely on what we are experiencing, trusting in the process we are going through, because it is a necessary step to open ourselves to the immense beauty of our Soul. Dealing with what we often do not understand is difficult and painful, but it is what is required for us to take the leap and land at our hidden side, which has been waiting for us for so long.

AWARENESS QUESTIONS

~ What transmutative processes are you going through?
~ Do you know the feeling of embracing grace after a phase of surrender and rebirth?
~ Do you allow yourself to trust the wait?

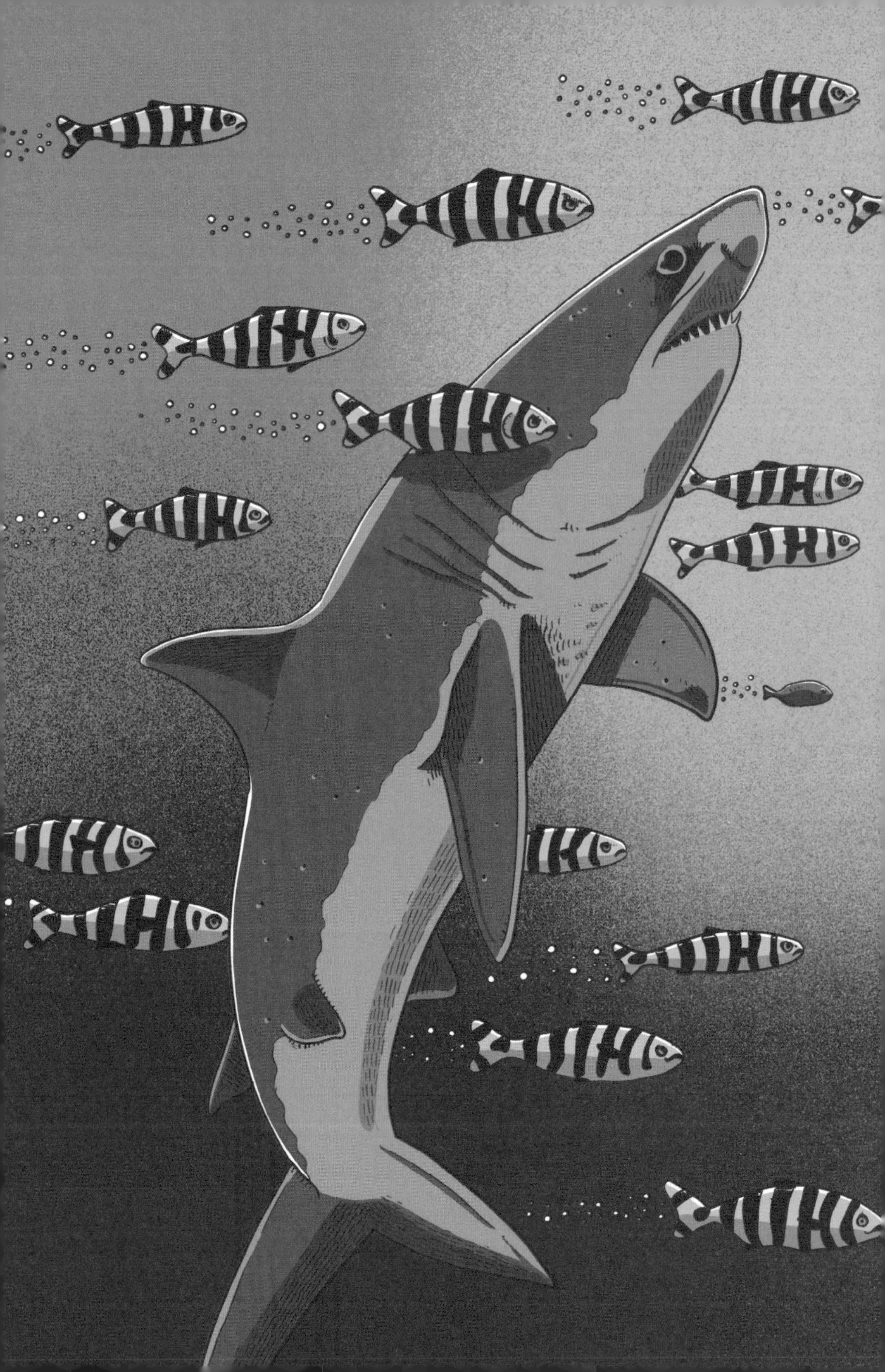

THE SHARK
The Predator of the Unconscious

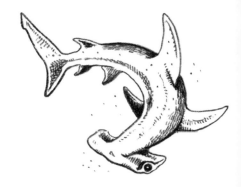

Portrayed in movies as a most dangerous monster, the Shark has forcibly entered the collective imaginary as a demon that lurks silently to launch bloody and unexpected attacks on anyone who intentionally or accidentally is swimming in its waters. This predator, which can measure from a few inches to several feet, can either be seen as an awesome or terrifying creature. Indeed, it still causes phobias and over time has become one of man's most hunted prey. Its appearance, with those sharp teeth, large mouth, and rapid body movements, make it an energetic, determined, calculating, stealthy,

> When you least expect it, I will emotionally ambush you to let you see, recognize, and heal your wounds.

aggressive, powerful, authoritative, and resilient animal. In Polynesia, Fiji, Hawaii, and Australia, several deities with Shark features are in charge of protecting places and their inhabitants. The Shark represents the predatory force of our unconscious mind: while apparently hindering us and making the moment of its arrival difficult, intense, and painful, in actual fact it is an ally who plays an uncomfortable role. It is the examiner with the task of making sure that we have learned the lessons from our previous experiences. When it appears, it is never pleasant: it often reveals past traumas that show us the emotional wounds that we have not yet seen or recognized. So it strongly drags us without letting go until we become aware of those wounds, until we decide to manage them, to reemerge renewed, leaving a worn-out pain under the sea.

AWARENESS QUESTIONS

~ How do you deal with yourself when old wounds come back to hurt?
~ Do you see a valuable ally in those who play this uncomfortable role with you, or do you become their predator in turn?
~ What are your phobias? Does the Shark fall among them?

133

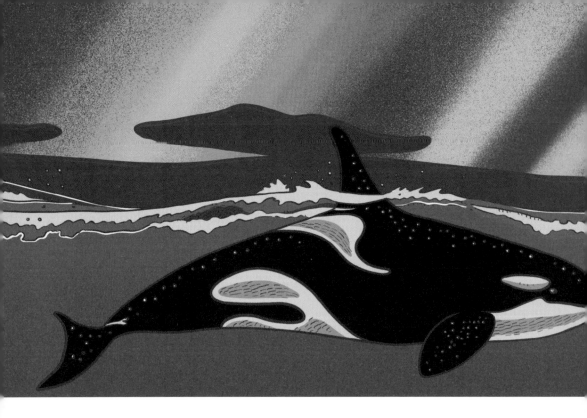

THE ORCA
The Family Lineage

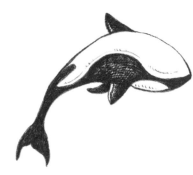

The Orca is the largest dolphin on the planet, a mammal that lives in matrifocal groups of different types. There are those that are sedentary, those that move from coast to coast, and those that undertake long-distance migrations in the open sea. Each group has its own complex hunting strategy, its own language (i.e., a dialect that is passed down from generation to generation), and each member participates in group activities, playing specific roles. Orcas are creative, playful, long-lived, and knowledgeable. They have a strong sense of community, express their affectivity in relationships, and cooperate for the success of the common goals of the entire family group. Seen as protectors and guardians of family traditions and lineages, according to the indigenous Kwakiutl nation of North America they were born from one of their ancestors who, during a whaling trip, was struck by lightning and fell into the sea and transformed into an Orca.

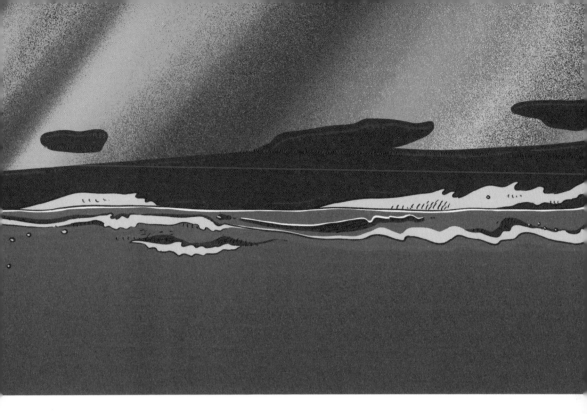

Orcas remind us that each of us comes from a complex, multi-faceted family system that, in every sphere of existence, has developed distinctive strategies and ways to survive and ensure its continuation. The family lineage from which we come is precious; it represents our roots; and if we know how to read and embrace it, it becomes an endless source of knowledge, wisdom, and strength, drawing from the experience of those who came before us.

Your roots hold all the power and knowledge of the force that has been passed down to you. Take care of them.

AWARENESS QUESTIONS

~ What is your relationship with your family lineage?
~ Are the knowledge and experience passed down by your ancestors valuable to you, or do you feel they are deeply limiting?
~ What is your relationship with traditions?

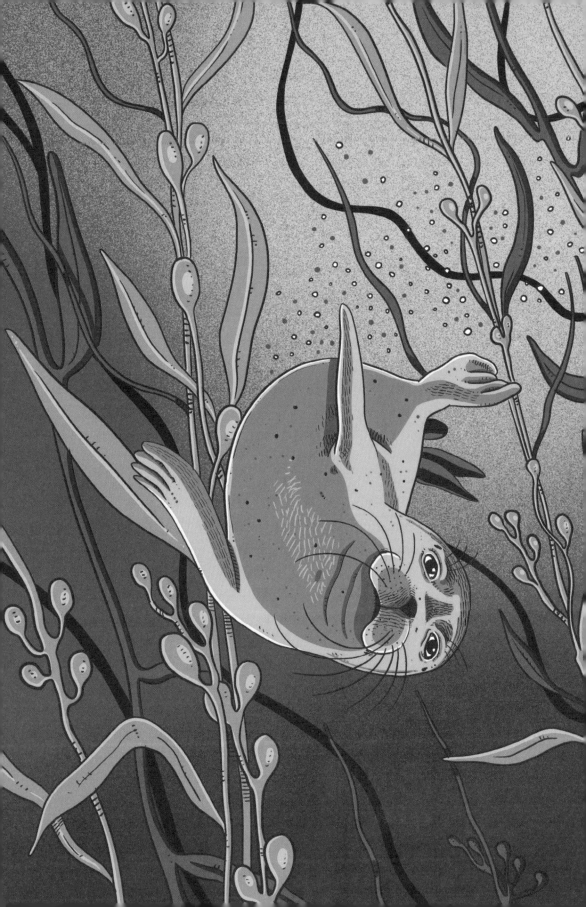

THE SEAL
The Benefits of Duality

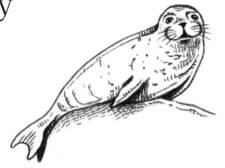

I n myths from Ireland, Iceland, and Scotland, Seals are believed to be women who have worn a special skin for millennia, thanks to which they live underwater. If necessary, they can remove it to walk in their human bodies on land. They are called Selkies and represent the link to the deep and wild nature of the feminine. As much as patriarchal power represses this side of them and Selkies try to fit into socially accepted archetypal female forms, an atavistic and irrepressible call connected to their being Seals always brings them back to the sea. Their desire to wear the ancient skins never wanes, and their marine families call them back to their homes underwater. At the same time,

when they feel the need, they allow themselves to strip off that magical shell and return to the land, exploring their earthly femininity. Interestingly enough, Seals are still hunted precisely for their skins. These incredible mammals live somewhere between Water and Earth, and have adapted to both environments, each serving different purposes. They thus represent the possibility of experiencing and living the dual aspect of existence, the ability to develop approaches and qualities to fully enjoy all that is inside and outside of us. They invite us to explore the possibilities offered by swimming in our deep waters and walking on the dry land, and to live both lives to the fullest, thus improving our health and well-being.

> Each of us has an above- and underground nature. It is healthy to explore and live both.

AWARENESS QUESTIONS

~ What happens to you when you dive into your deep waters? What do you feel?
~ Same question about when you enjoy the warm rays of light on your dry land.
~ How do you deal with the duality inherent in every aspect of life?

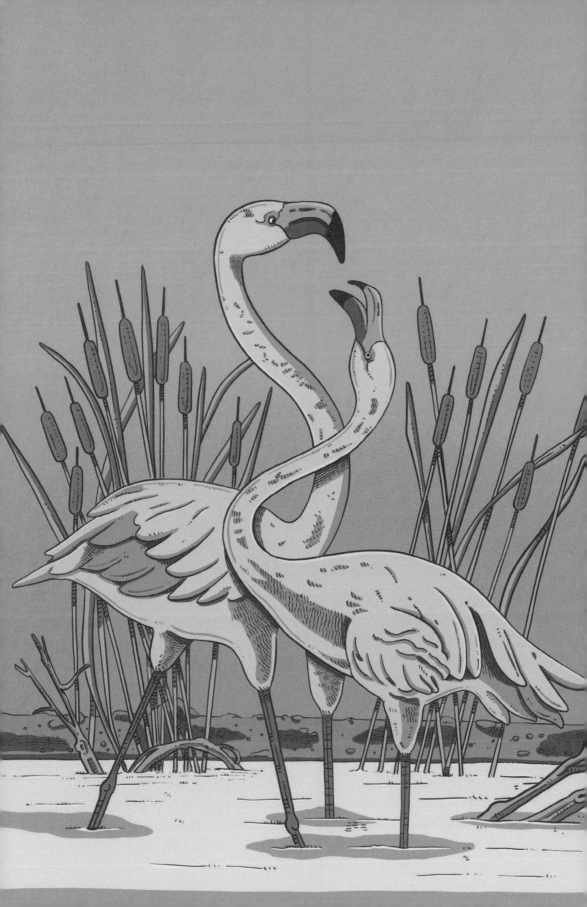

THE FLAMINGO
The Elegant Equilibrist

The name Flamingo means "red-winged," and it is its singular color that amazes anyone who crosses this wonderful waterbird's path. The bright pink of its feathers evokes unconditional love, total openness of the Heart, but also maternal, romantic love that heals us with its gentle, tender, and affectionate embrace. For Flamingos, this color in its bright, vibrant, and saturated hue indicates good health, vigor, and fertility. There are also red and white-colored species, and this variation is due to the different diet. Slender and majestic, tireless fliers, friendly, and long-lived, Flamingos live in colonies and are skilled dancers and equilibrists. They, in fact, sleep and rest on one leg, and are often seen with their long necks completely submerged in the water of salt lakes, which they choose as their habitat between one migration and another. They represent the ability to live in perfect balance, to find a pivot around which to take roots. The Flamingo is the purity of love that expands from within, allowing one to seek simplicity, beauty, and sharing. The color pink symbolizes the strength of the unconstrained Heart that generously gives, spreads its wings, and flies high as a spiritual harbinger of freedom and pleasure. The Flamingo invites us to constantly, elegantly dance between extremes, to feel the profound sense of justice and order that balance gives us.

Learn to elegantly dance
with the balance,
find your pivot,
and, from it, spread the pure
love that will make you fly.

AWARENESS QUESTIONS

~ Are you a balanced person? Or do you love excess?
~ How do you feel when you perceive yourself in balance?
~ Does offering and spreading your love give you the feeling of taking flight?

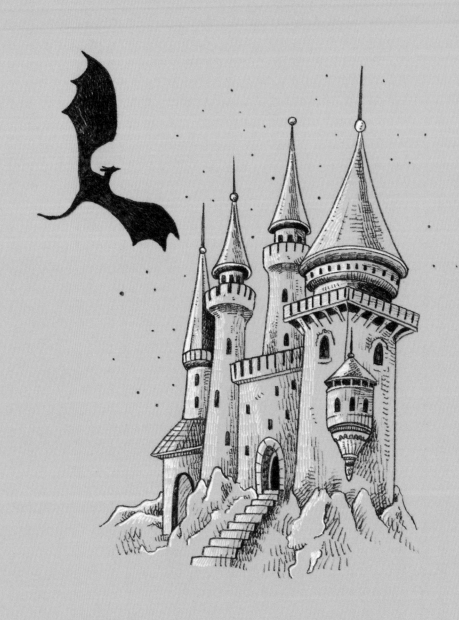

IMAGINARY ANIMALS

The Imaginary Animals come to remind us that we are made of magic. They tell us that our very existence is a mystery, a miracle, that we need to make room for the invisible, to what is not demonstrable or logically explainable. Their very existence nurtures the fantasy and imagination of the inner child within each of us, gives us joy and lightheartedness, and expands our horizons, making us open to the dreamlike, fairylike, magical worlds that they embody. They bring back that sparkle, which every child knows well, to our adult eyes.

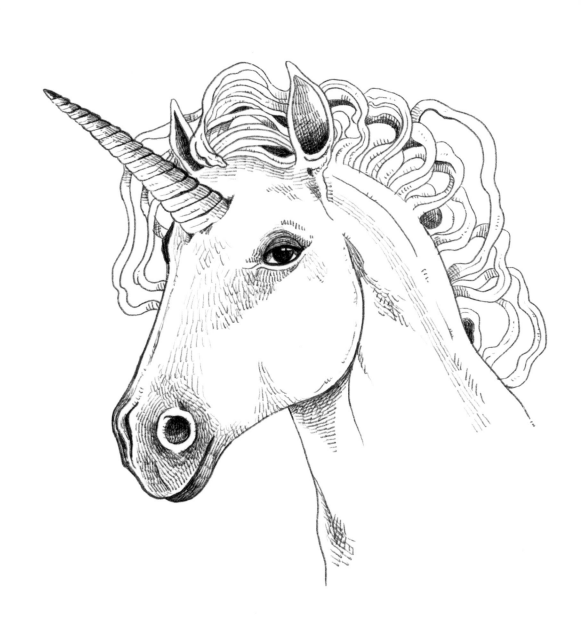

THE UNICORN
The Spiritual Purity

Inhabitants of very high spiritual dimensions, Unicorns are mythical creatures that throughout the ages have represented purity, spiritual elevation, immortality, and truth. Considered magical, infallible healers, bearers of high frequencies, of vibrations of pure love, Unicorns appear as white horses with a large twisted, spiraling horn in the center of their foreheads and a rainbow-hued tail. Their magic is associated with the transmutative power of the rainbow and the white light that, containing all colors of the spectrum, holds all their potential and combinations. In the Middle Ages, their horn was believed to heal everything and protect against all poisons, so the Vikings traded narwhal horns at great

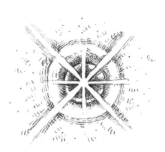

> You are pure light, wearing the forms of all colors to experience yourself through matter. Honor your spiritual purity.

expense, passing them off as those of Unicorns. The message this creature conveys to us is to honor our sacredness, spiritual purity, and luminous truth that no human experience, no matter how terrible, can extinguish. The Unicorn tells us that we are multidimensional beings, vibrating on various levels of consciousness, and invites us to reach that of the Spirit. The Unicorn is mentioned in medieval Romance literature, in Renaissance volumes and paintings, and in the Bible and in Pliny the Elder's *Naturalis Historia*. They are currently beloved and popular characters in Western pop culture.

AWARENESS QUESTIONS

~ Do Unicorns populate your imagination? What do they represent to you?
~ Do you feel that the purity of your Spirit cannot be damaged by anything?
~ Do you use practices or techniques to reach higher frequencies?

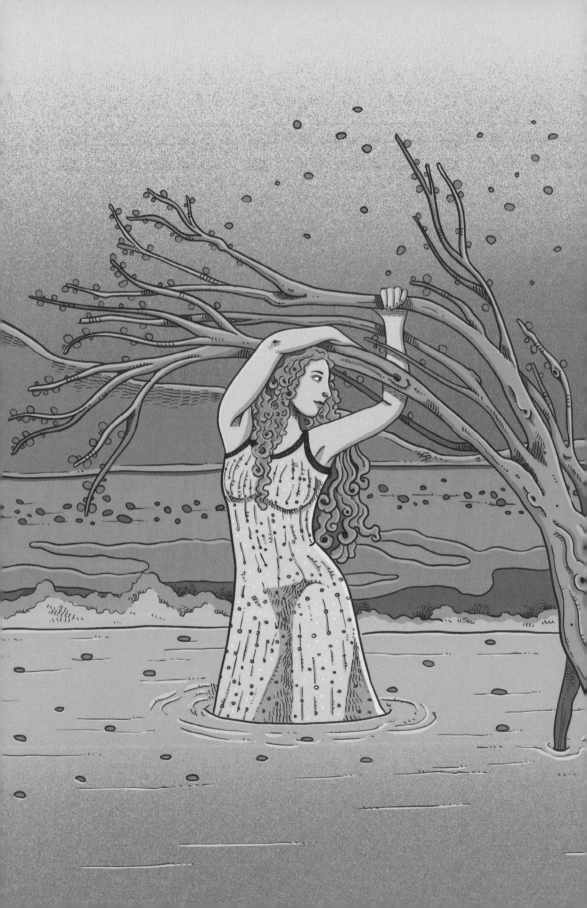

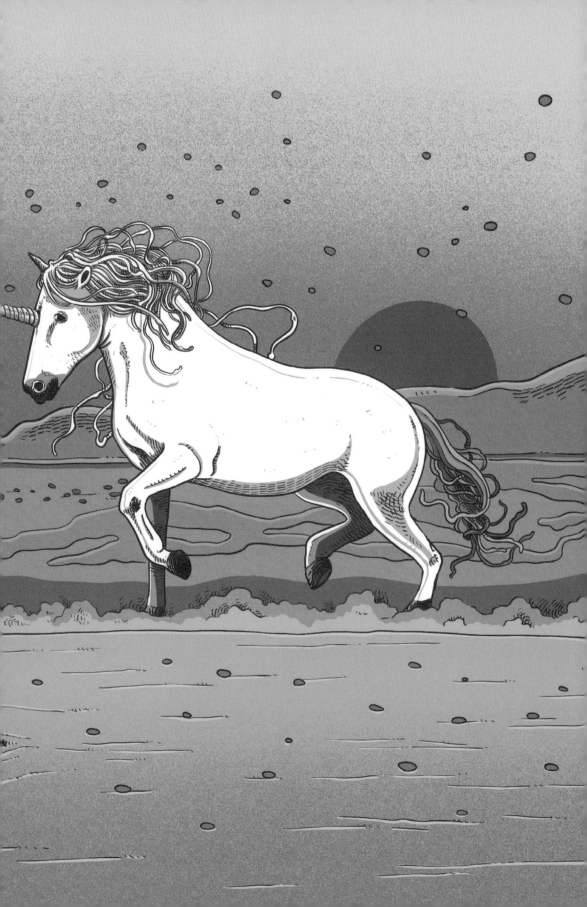

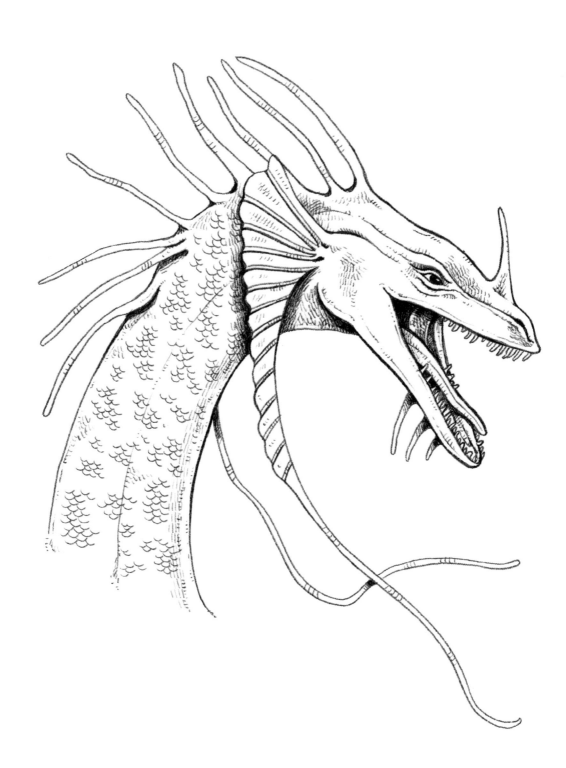

THE DRAGON
The Guardian of the Treasure

Demonic and angelic at the same time, the Dragon is the initiatory creature guarding the treasure, that which only great heroes can get, precisely by defeating the Dragon itself. As ancient as the Universe, wise and ruthless, this creature dominates and wields the power of the four elements. It inhabits the heavens, the deep waters, and the hidden lands, and possesses the blazing power of fire. It protects the gifts of the Soul and at once represents its darkest and most impenetrable mental faculties. To touch it is to access another level of knowledge and awareness. You will never be the same when you meet it, for you will have crossed a threshold

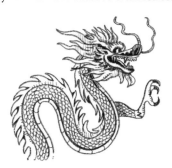

> To get the treasure, you need to unleash your inner hero. Only the bold and daring can defeat me.

that will immensely expand your inner self and horizons. The Dragon teaches us that what is as precious as a treasure must be gained, earned, and pursued. It invites us not to stop in the face of obstacles that will stand between us and our treasure, because only by testing ourselves can we understand whether we are really interested in our goal, or it is just a whim not worth fighting for. In Eastern cultures, especially in China and Japan, the Dragon is regarded as a divine being that bestows good luck, success, and prosperity. It embodies the forces of nature and imperial power.

AWARENESS QUESTIONS

~ Do you know how to be courageous and intrepid when you really want something?
~ Do you identify yourself as the Dragon, as the hero, or as the treasure?
~ Is there something fundamental that you want to achieve in this quest?
   What do you want to protect instead?
~ What are the treasures hidden inside you?

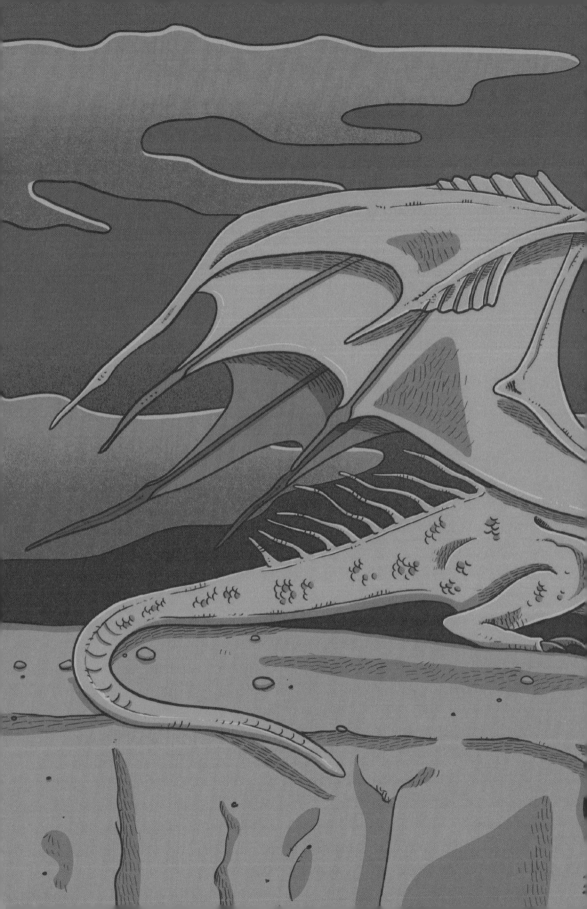

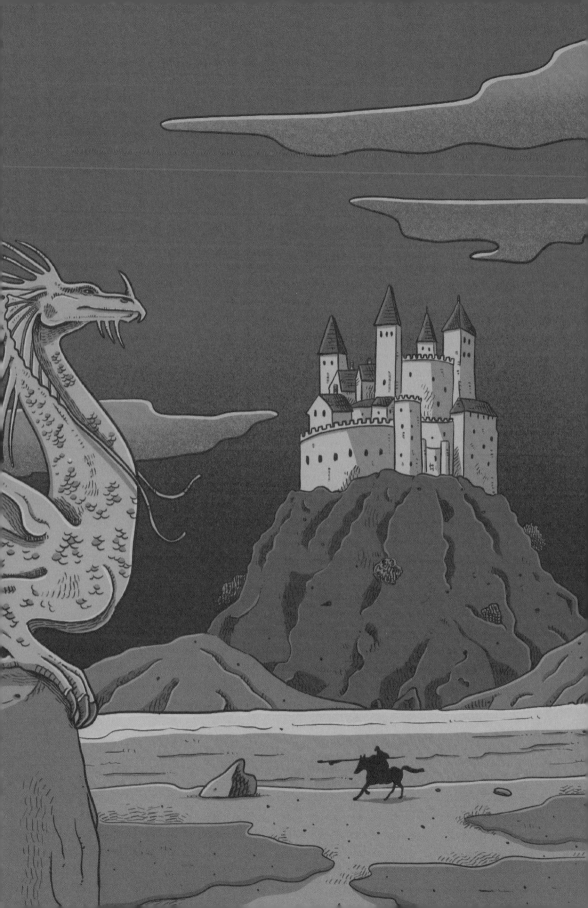

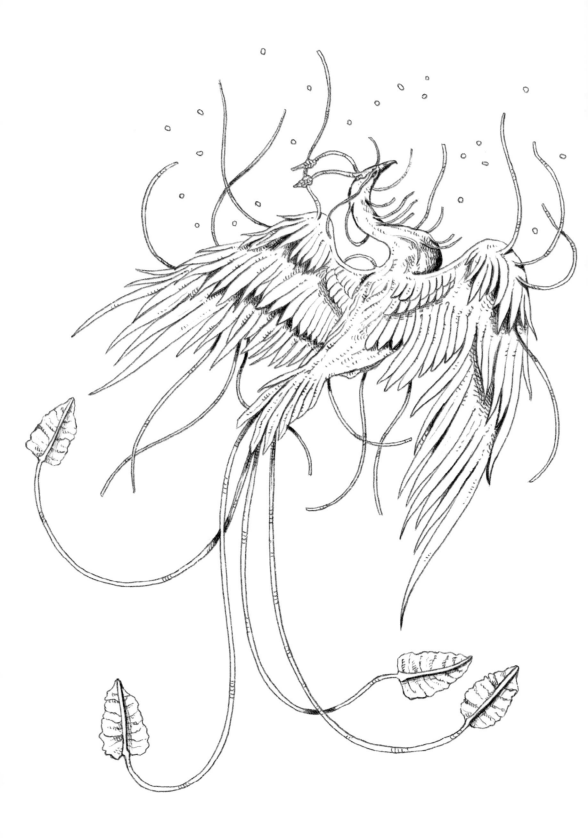

THE PHOENIX
Rising from its Ashes

The alchemical bird par excellence, in all myths the Phoenix is universally recognized as a symbol of resurrection, rebirth, and transformation. This process involves both physical death and all symbolic deaths experienced in Life. The Phoenix is the fierce red bird that is reborn from its own ashes, either in its egg or adult form, and represents the immortality of the Spirit. The Phoenix reminds us that, to be spiritually reborn, the parts that hinder our evolution must die and that sabotaging, repetitive thought patterns, and attitudes that prevent us from growing must be set on fire.

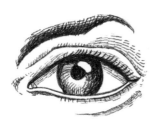

When all that you were is burned to ashes, from them may rise an unexpected version of you.

All unfruitful things must be left aside, egoic attachments must be destroyed, and victimhood must be dissolved. To rise again, we must always die; and if we do not accept this, death becomes painful. If we instead accept this truth, rebirth and evolution are ensured. We must interiorize this message and remember it especially in moments of pain and suffering. Invoke the power of the Phoenix when you are going through a difficult time to overcome it, illuminated by the light of the new you that is already there, awaiting you on the other side.

AWARENESS QUESTIONS

~ How many times have you died and been reborn in this existence?
~ Symbolically, does the Phoenix represent you?
~ What do you need to burn to keep evolving?
~ In what new form do you want to rise?
~ Are you interested in evolving into a new version of you?

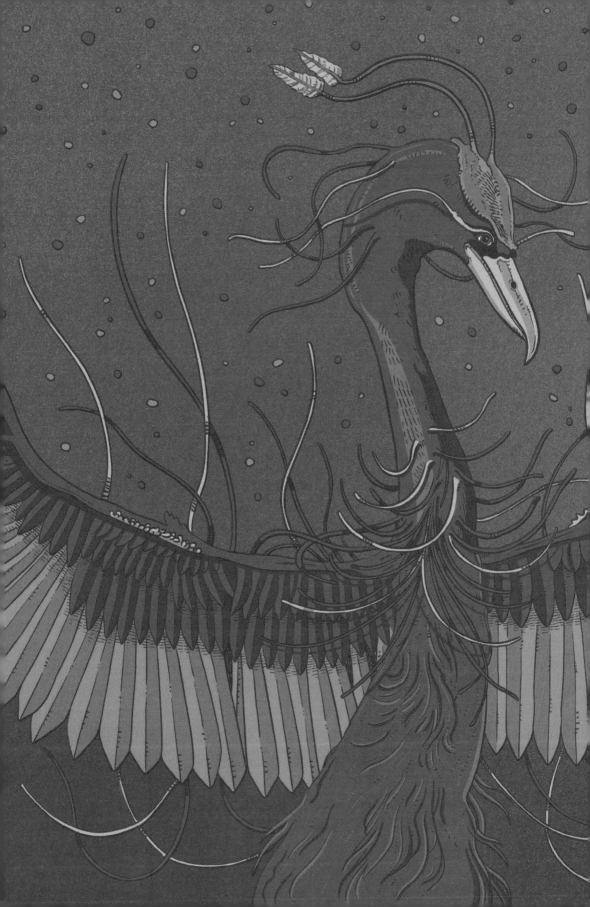

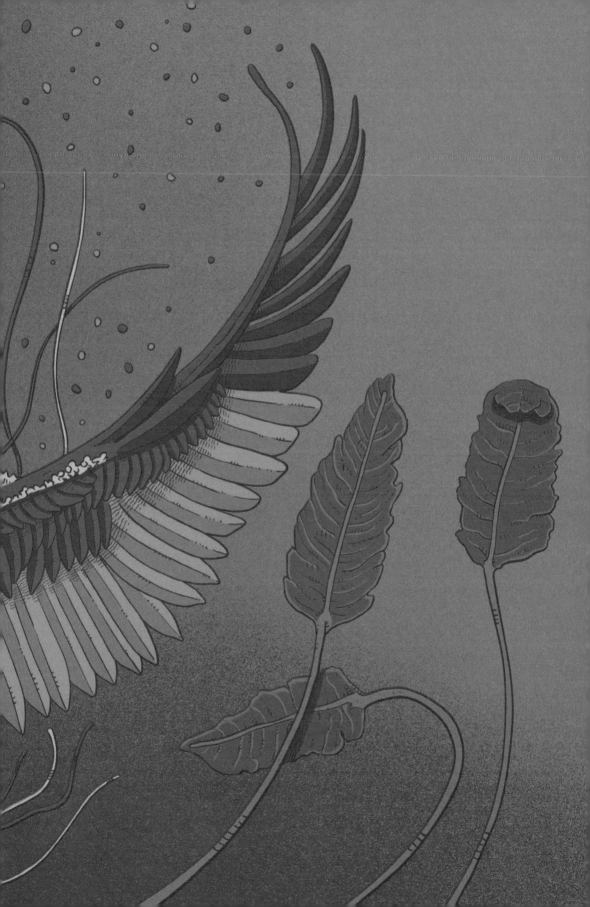

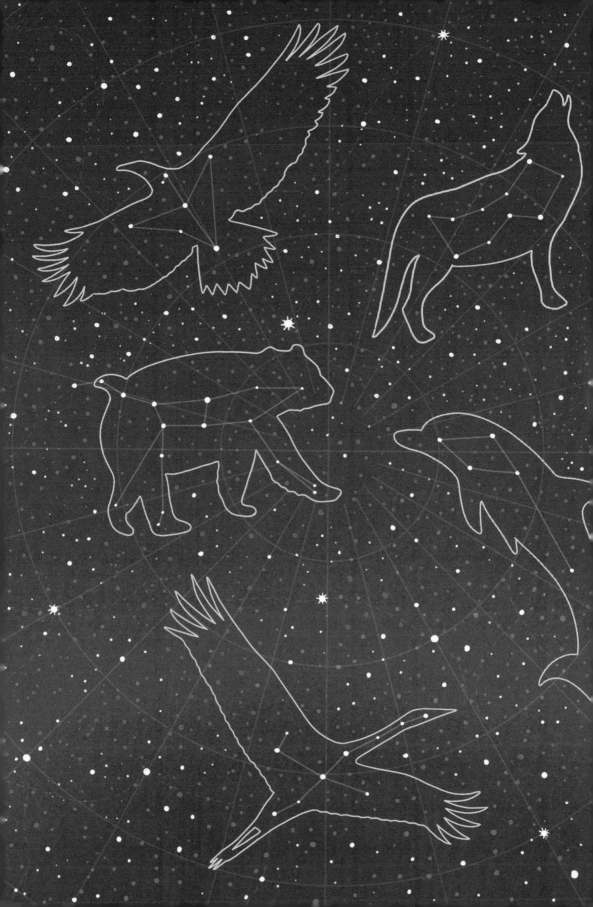

As you have seen, the teachings of the archetypal animals can be antithetical and convey conflicting—yet not mutually exclusive—concepts. Each of them, in fact, speaks to us at a specific time, and those that resonate with us at one time may not necessarily do it again at another. This is why some animal guides accompany us through the subtle world only as we walk certain paths and then, once we reach our destination, say goodbye, giving way to others. It is up to you, aware of your needs in the present moment, to choose which familiar to invoke. What do you need right now? What resources, what medicine do you need? Healing Animals come and show themselves through dreams; we pass them on the street; they populate our imagination. We can meet them in visualizations, shamanic journeys, or any other practice we use to connect with our inner self. If we are able to give them a face and listen to their voice, the journey together will become conscious and very interesting. Which animal do you feel accompanied by? Because it's true, various members of our spiritual tribe travel with us depending on the moment, but don't forget that the tribe leader accompanies you forever and will be by your side from birth to death. We can usually recognize it by instinct, because in its nature we see our own reflected. By mirroring ourselves in the animals recounted here and in all those that populate our psyche, we can get to know ourselves in a fun, yet profound, way. I hope this book has helped you to identify them better. Thank you all for your time and dedication.

NOTES

BIOGRAPHIES

KIKOSMICA (FEDERICA ZIZZARI)

Federica is a Soul Curandera, an alchemist of the heart. A certified holistic practitioner, Family Constellation facilitator, spiritual artist, channeler, Akashic Records reader, and Soul Coach, she works in the field of counseling to guide anyone who wants to find a balance in Life, turning wounds into resourceful, blooming opportunities. She designs individual and group paths of Inner Growth. She has drawn the "Carte divinatorie degli Alberi Sacri" (Divining Cards of Sacred Trees) and wrote the book *Messaggi Angelici* (Angelic Messages). Her artistic and spiritual research is constantly evolving, always at the service of Love and Life.

GIADA UNGREDDA

Giada is an Italian illustrator and graphic designer. She is passionate for fantasy and steampunk novels and has always imagined fictional worlds. She has been drawing for as long as she can remember, and in her spare time she writes stories and illustrates them with watercolors, pencils, and nibs. Since 2020, she has been producing botanical and educational illustrated plates for outreach projects.